EAR
The Switchboard of Your Body

EAR
The Switchboard of Your Body

Rama Venkataraman
(M.D. Acupuncture)
Indian Academy of Acupuncture Science

Srikunj Sadbhavana Manch
New Delhi

Cataloging in Publication Data — DK

[Courtesy: D.K. Agencies (P) Ltd. <docinfo@dkagencies.com>]

Venkataraman, Rama, author.
Ear : the switchboard of your body / Rama Venkataraman. (M.D. Acupuncture).
pages cm
Reprint of revised edition: 2012.
ISBN 9788182650213 (PBK)

1. Ear – Anatomy. 2. Ear – Diseases – Treatment. 3. Ear – Care and hygiene. 4. Ear – Acupuncture. I. Title.

LCC QM507.V46 2022 | DDC 611.85 23

ISBN 978-81-8265-021-3 (PBK)

First published in 2002
Revised edition published in 2012
First reprint 2021
Second reprint 2023

Published and printed by:
Srikunj Sadbhavana Manch
"Srikunj", F-52, Bali Nagar
New Delhi - 110015

Distributed by:
D.K. Printworld (P) Ltd.
Regd. office : "Vedaśrī", F-395, Sudarshan Park
(Metro Station: ESI Hospital) New Delhi - 110015
Phones : (011) 25453975, 25466019
E-mail: indology@dkprintworld.com
Web: www.dkprintworld.com

From the Author

AURICULOTHERAPY wherein the whole body is treated in a single appendage — the Ear — had fascinated me from the time I was introduced to it some years back. Further visible clear proof of it came when I used it on the patients and started getting instant results.

My experience has been compounded with other professionals in the field like Prof. Dr P.B. Lohiya and Prof. Dr Anton Jayasuriya and other colleagues of mine who had been reporting excellent therapeutic results by stimulating ear points either by needle or by other ingenious methods like applying seeds, electronic point finder and stimulator machines or simple massage.

This is a most simplistic, effective, natural mode of treatment and is within the reach of every human being. I felt if this system be popularised and modalities of treatment understood clearly, it can be of immense benefit and an answer for the multitude of suffering humanity.

This in fact was an ancient system of cure used in the Eastern countries like China, Japan, Korea and to some extent in India too many centuries ago. Here we are only reviving the old knowledge.

This book is a humble endeavour to present the information with clarity and with a number of easy-to-understand diagrams.

Accepting the information with open mind will without fail augur results. I always tell my students if human mind can invent a remote to work the T.V., is it not possible for the Almighty to give us a remote in the Ear to operate the body?

I was assisted in my work by Mr Malik in computer graphics and in drawings by artist Mr S.D. Shellar and Mr Chandrashekhar Patil. The proofreading work was assisted by Mrs Radha Bhat. The cover design was assisted by Mr Niraj Chaturvedi.

In this endeavour of mine I got my inspiration from my students who showed keen interest in knowing the Ear therapeutics. I dedicate this to my students and patients who have been my constant source of inspiration in understanding this subtle science — a God-given gift for the welfare of humanity.

Dr Rama Venkataraman
e-mail: <ramavenkataraman75@gmail.com>
website: <www.acupuncturebyrama.com

Introduction

OUR body is replete with wonders. The intricate working of the body mechanism is not easy to grapple and understand for laymen and scientists alike. If all the riddles of the body can be understood by dissection, analysis, and logic alone then all the health problems of the body would have been long before solved and our cities won't be crammed with so many medicos, hospitals, and scientists with their health potions eternally trying to find answers to our health problems. However, if we turn our antenna slightly and take a note of our body's own mechanism of healing itself, we would be lot more benefited.

Have you ever wondered when you press your palm, finger as well as the body surface, there are certain parts which are more tender and painful in comparison to others? These are the response points in our body. They are the body's unique signal mechanism giving us the message, that a corresponding part inside the body is not in working order. If we only take the cue and understand the body language we will have diagnosis and the cure within our reach, a mechanism of cure much simpler and easy to use than applying human logic to every problem and solve it by pills and vials. Further these points act as a fine-tuning control mechanism gearing the body to ideal health as it starts slipping, akin to a stitch in time saving nine. Thus these tender signalling points act as a preventive control saving the body from slipping to any severe lapse in its upkeep.

It would be wonderful if people get a working knowledge of the sensitive points designed by nature and understand their relations to the vital organs of our body to keep themselves in perpetual good health.

Among the signal points in the body ear has a unique place. Ear with its numerous nerve endings is a very sensitive part of the anatomy. In the ear, body is represented in an upside down position like the child in the womb. Ear being a small area it is easily accessible and well responds to treatment. Many countries around the globe are getting wise to this mode of healing the body, that is, stimulating the corresponding ear points for improving the body's working. Here is the opportunity for us to learn and understand as to how ear acts as the switchboard of the body.

Contents

1

Ear
The Reflector of Your Body

OUR body has a unique mechanism of reflecting its working in various parts of our body. The internal organs whose access and working is difficult to make out from outside give subtle signals along certain exposed parts of our body indicating its working. Thus we have hand-foot reflexology, the meridian therapy, the head, nose and ear reflexology.

Of all these the ear reflexology has a prime place in diagnosing and healing our body, the reason being ear is one of the most sensitive organs. It is supplied by a rich network of nerves bringing in and taking out information to various parts of our body. Our ear hence acts like a sensitive radar.

Important Nerve and Blood Supply to Ear

Some of the important nerve supplies to the ear are:

1. Temporo-auricular nerve
2. Great Auricular nerve
3. Cranial nerves —
   (i) Trigeminal (fifth cranial nerve) —
   Supply to muscles and skin of face and jaws.

   (ii) Glossopharyngeal (ninth cranial nerve) —
   Supply to muscles of palate, throat, tongue, salivary glands.

   (iii) Vagus (tenth cranial nerve) —
   Supply to muscles of throat, larynx, heart, lungs, abdominal organs.

(iv) Occipital
Supply sensation to back of neck, ear and scalp

(v) Facial (seventh cranial nerve)
Supply muscles of face and facial expression

4. Sympathetic and para sympathetic fibres.

Apart from the nerves ear also has a rich supply of blood from branches of important arteries and veins.

Some of the important blood supplies to the body are:

ARTERIES

1. Meningeal artery — from brain
2. Tympanic artery — connected to internal ear
3. Auricular arteries
   (i) Deep auricular artery
   (ii) Posterior auricular artery
   (iii) Superficial auricular artery
4. Temporal artery of external carotid artery
5. Artery of the pterygoid canal

VEINS

Venous drainage occurs in:

1. Superficial temporal vein
2. External jugular vein, and
3. Mastoid vein

LYMPH NODES

1. Posterior auricular lymph nodes
2. Posterior lymph nodes
3. Mastoid lymph nodes
4. Spinal lymph nodes
5. Pre-tragic lymph nodes
6. Anterior lymph nodes

The pathology of different internal organs is mirrored in

the ear which then responds accurately to stimulation, passing the impulses to the organ concerned bringing in a cure.

There are more than 200 reflex points in the ear.

Important Reflex Points of the Ear

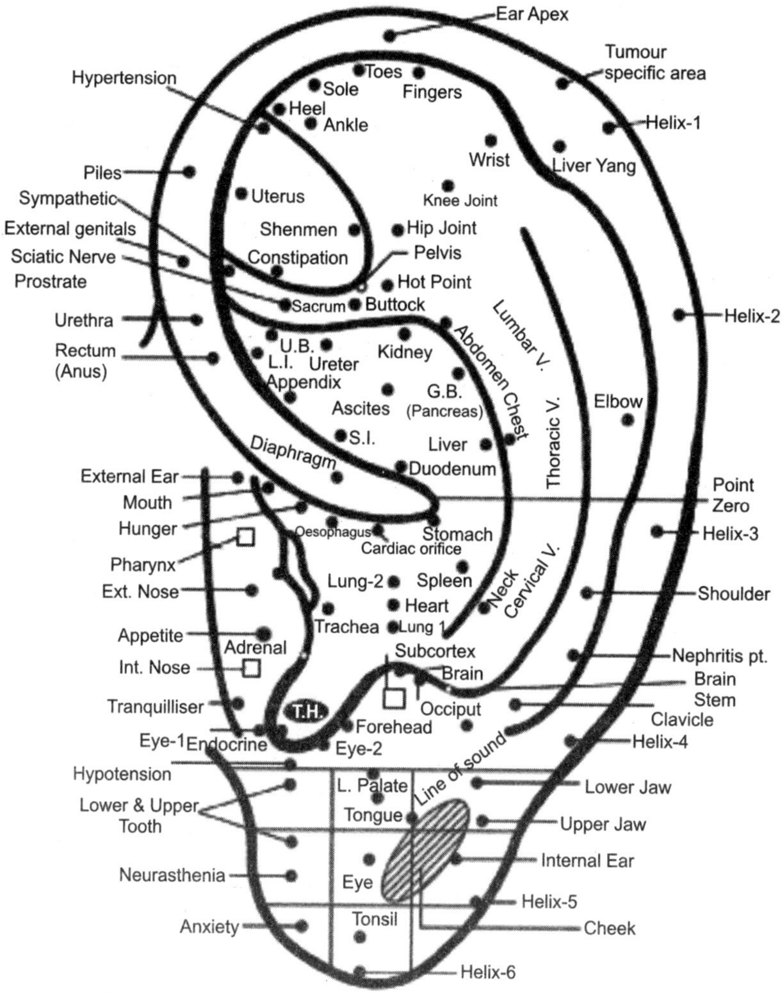

☐ Parts along the inner side

Ear points are most useful to:

1. Control pain
2. To cure internal organ disorder
3. In drug and alcohol addiction
4. Acupuncture anaesthesia

The science of healing body by ear stimulation was well known in India at ancient times. In Vedic literature there is a treatise called *Suchi chikitsa* where the ear is mentioned as a important part for curing the body. Our ancient customs of piercing the ear and wearing golden and silver studs and rings have a clear connection in using ear for bringing in cure of the body. In children ear-piercing is done both to stimulate vitality and provide immunity. This science was also well understood and developed in China.

North Africa and certain Middle East countries were using extensively ear-piercing for curing acute sciatic pain and other problems traditionally and in present times too. Of late Western countries are realising the significance of ear stimulation. France especially has gone much ahead in using this science. The Nogier School of Ear Acupuncture in France and Munich Auriculotherapy Association have contributed lately in understanding and spreading Auriculotherapy.

Our ear can be equated to the switchboard of our body. The internal lesions in the organs like gastric ulcer etc. are immediately reflected in the ear. In China at the Institute of Physiology in Shanghai several experiments were conducted to show how internal changes in the organs are flashed immediately in the ear. As the body situation improves ear pathology also shows improvements. Thus the corresponding ear points act as radar increasing and decreasing in response accordingly.

Representation of the Body in the Ear

The body lies in the ear like a child in a mother's womb. The head lies below in the earlobe while the legs lie curled up in the upper portion.

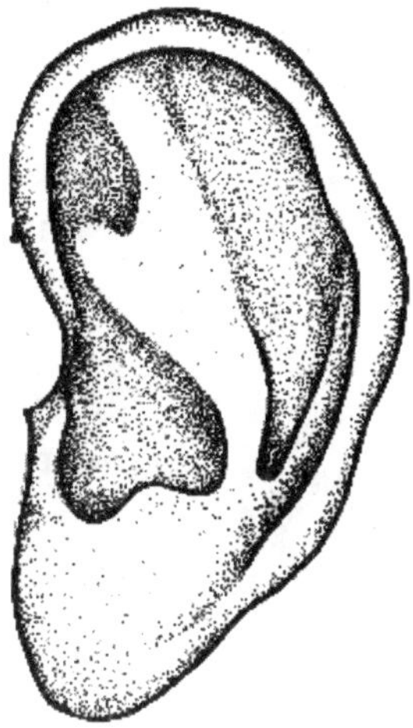

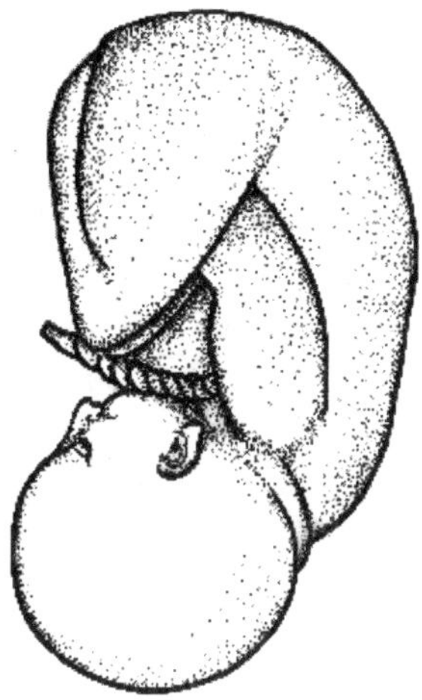

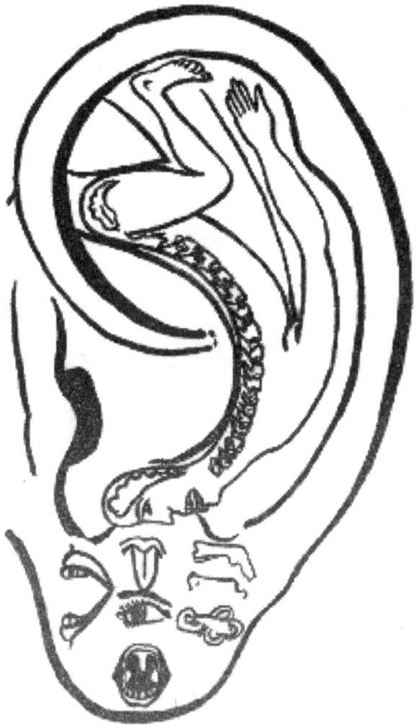

Human Body Representation in the Ear

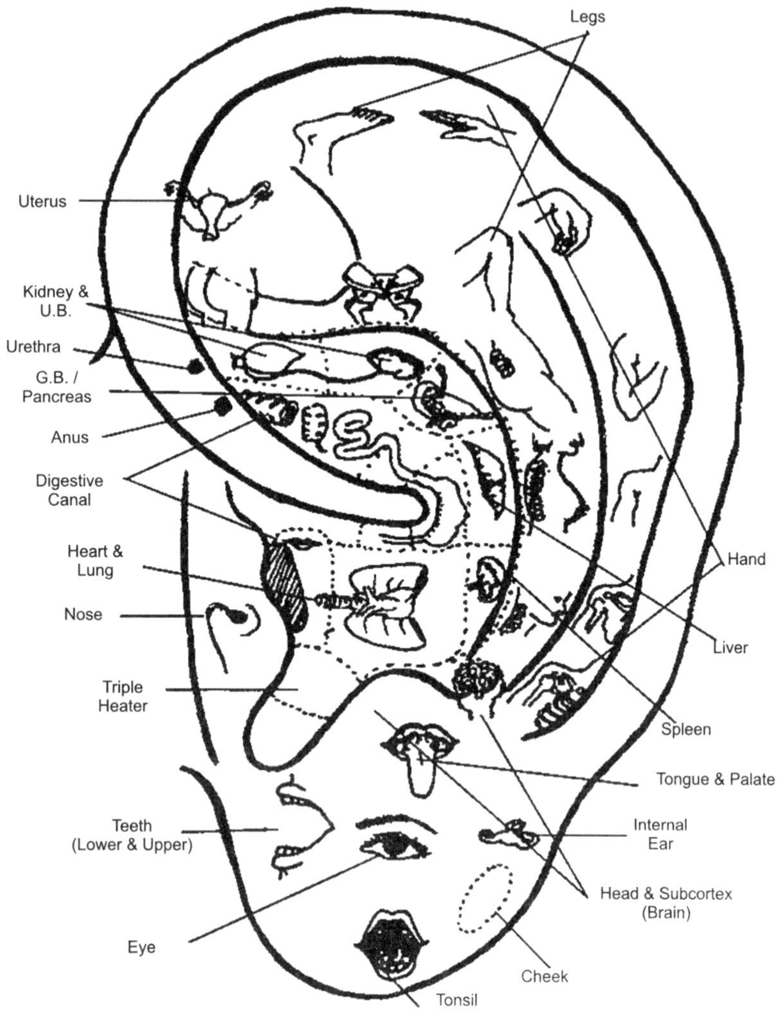

Structure of the Ear

An understanding of the structure of the ear will greatly help in knowing the location of different organs of the body in the ear.

On examining the structure of the ear we can notice two important features. One, an outer surface shaped like a question mark and an inside concave portion divided into two by a protruding cartilage.

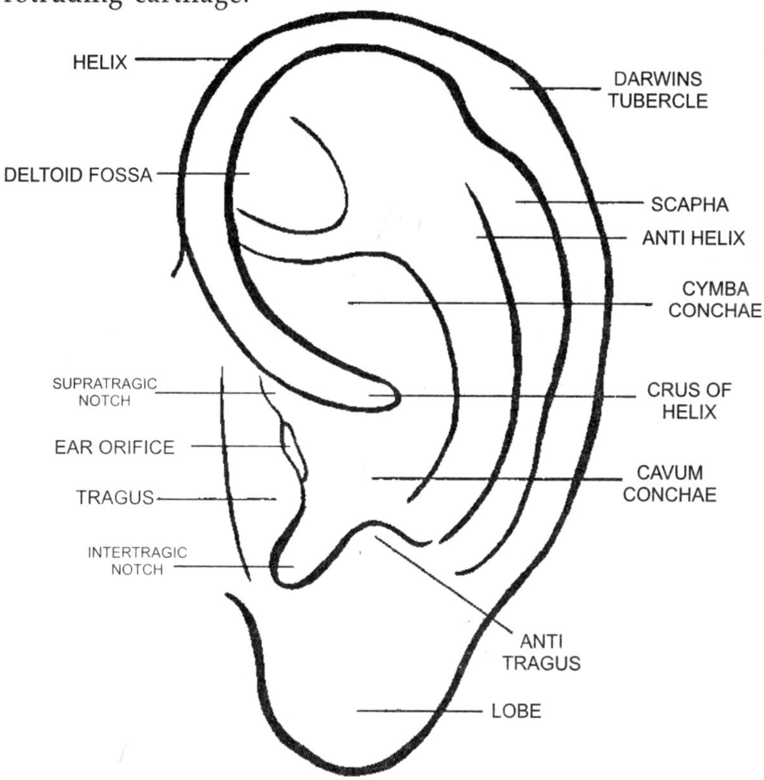

The outer portion consists of

1. Helix — It is the outer rim of the ear which takes a turn and enters the concave cavity as the crus of helix.
2. Scapha — Next to helix, a flat surface.
3. Antihelix — Next to scapha again shaped like a rim which divides in the upper part into two branches,

namely: superior crus of anti-helix and inferior crus of anti-helix.

4. Deltoid Fossa — A depression between two crura of anti-helix triangular in shape.

5. Anti Tragus — The lower portion of the ear has two flaps just above the earlobe on either side of the ear orifice. The one along the anti-helix is in the outer side and is called anti-tragus.

6. Tragus — The flap opposite to anti-tragus along the cheek is called tragus.

The inner concave portion has two main parts:

1. Cymba conchae : The upper concave cavity.
2. Cavum conchae : The lower concave cavity.

Both the cavities are divided by tapering point of the crus of helix.

Further the cavum conchae has two notches:

Inter-tragic notch: Along the lower end of the ear orifice between tragus and anti-tragus.

Supra-tragic notch: Along the upper end of the ear orifice along the face.

Earlobe: It is the lower portion of the ear without a cartilage. A soft portion lying free below the ear structure.

Back of the Ear:It is the yang surface of the ear. It has a prominent groove.

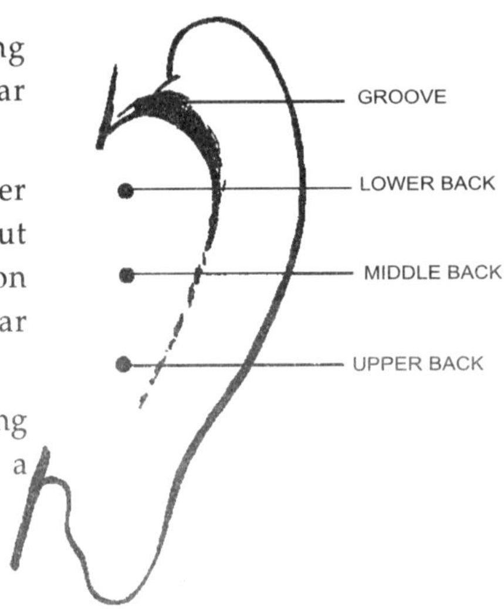

2

Representation of the Body Parts

In the ear the human body is represented in an upside position as in human foetus. The bottom portion of the ear, the lobe represents the face, the rest of the body lies in a curled up position with the back of the body, the brain, neck, spinal column lying along the outer portion of the ear while the internal organs like stomach, liver, spleen, kidney, heart and lungs lie internally along the inner concave region. The ear is made of cartilage and soft tissue.

The Earlobe

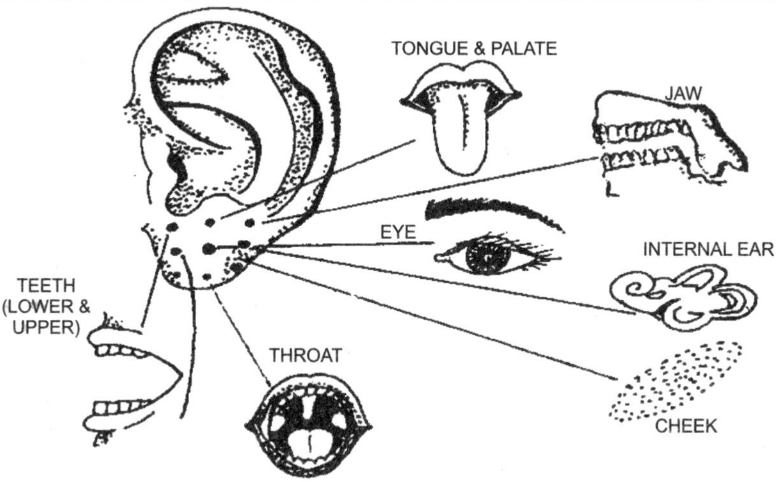

The Earlobe

This represents the face area till the forehead. The lobe can be divided into nine parts with two vertical and three horizontal lines.

REPRESENTATION

1. In the centre lies the eye.
2. Above eye lie lower palate and tongue.
3. Below eye lie upper palate, throat and tonsils.
4. To the right next to eye lies the internal ear.
5. Above the ear lie the jaws.
6. To the left along the face lie the lower and upper teeth.

L.1 Lower teeth

☞ Severe toothache.

L.4 Upper teeth

☞ Severe toothache. The teeth area on electro stimulation produces anaesthetic effect, can be used for tooth extraction.

L.2 Tongue and palate

☞ Lesion in tongue, ulcer in palate.

L.3 Jaw

☞ Dislocation of jaw, lock jaw, mumps, arthritis of the jaw bone.

L.5 Eye

☞ Eye disease — conjunctivitis, myopia and other eye problems.

L.6 Inner ear

☞ Hearing difficulty, equilibrium, nerve deafness, vertigo, travel sickness.

L.8 Throat:

☞ Tonsillitis, pharyngitis, laryngitis.

L.9 Cheek area

☞ Sub-mucus fibrosis, pigmentation of face, wrinkles, facial paralysis, Trigeminal neurolgia, Bell's palsy.

The lobe also represents cerebral cortex of brain consisting of cerebellum and cortex as shown in figure.

Cerebellum

☞ Activating this helps in motor co-ordination, spasms, relieves tremors, vertigo, equilibrium, depression.

Cortex

☞ Consists of occipital, temporal, parietal, frontal and prefrontal lobes.

Occipital	:	Helps in visual disorders — blindness.
Temporal	:	Helps in auditory disorders.
Parietal	:	Helps in relieving pain, migraine, etc.
Frontal	:	Helps in curing paralysis, improves motor action.
Pre-frontal	:	Helps in decision-making. Improves concentration, brings down worry, nervousness.

Master Cerebral

👂 Found below the tooth area.

☞ Represents pre-frontal lobe and part of cerebral cortex.

☞ Helps in making conscious decision.

☞ Diminishes nervous anxiety, fear, worry, obsessive compulsive disorder, pessimistic thinking, psychosomatic disorders.

Master Sensorial

- Found at the same point as eye point in the lobe.
- Controls sensory cerebral cortex of parietal lobe.
- Reduces unpleasant excessive sensation.
- Diminishes tingling sensation, ringing in ears, blurred vision.

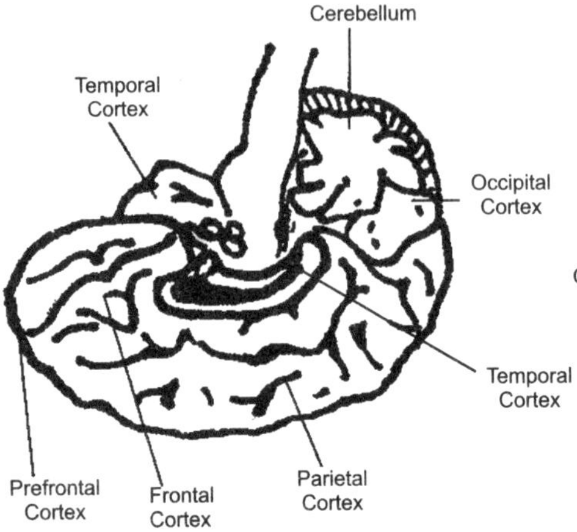

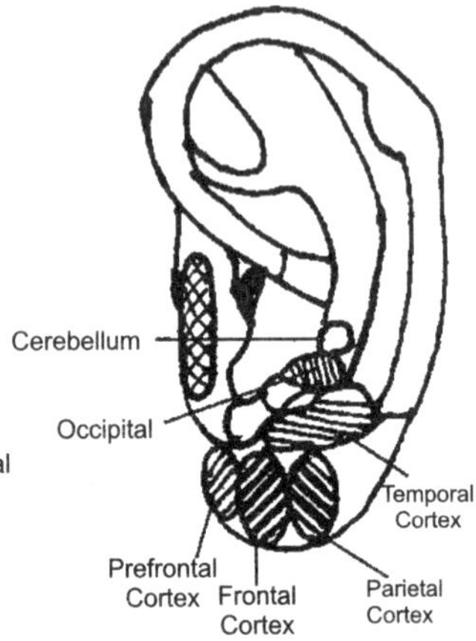

The Anti-Helix and Anti-Tragus

The anti-tragus and anti-helix correspond to the neck area, spine till coccyx.

1. The forehead and occiput area lies in the anti-tragus.
2. The subcortex lies in the inner wall of the anti-tragus.
3. Brain point lies in the junction of anti-tragus and anti-helix.
4. Extending along the rim of the anti-helix are the neck, thoracic and lumbar vertebrae.
5. The buttock, hip joint and thigh lie in the inferior crus of the anti-helix.
6. The foot, ankle the lower limb lie in the superior crus of anti-helix.
7. The knee in the junction of the two crura.

Anti-tragus

This represents the head area. In the outside are the forehead and occiput area. In the inner side is the subcortex region of the brain.

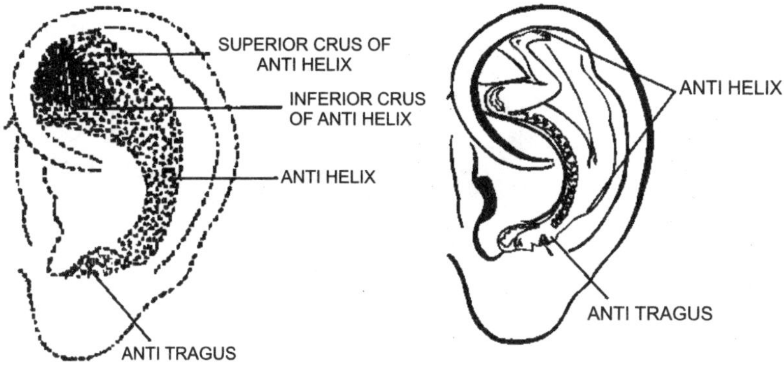

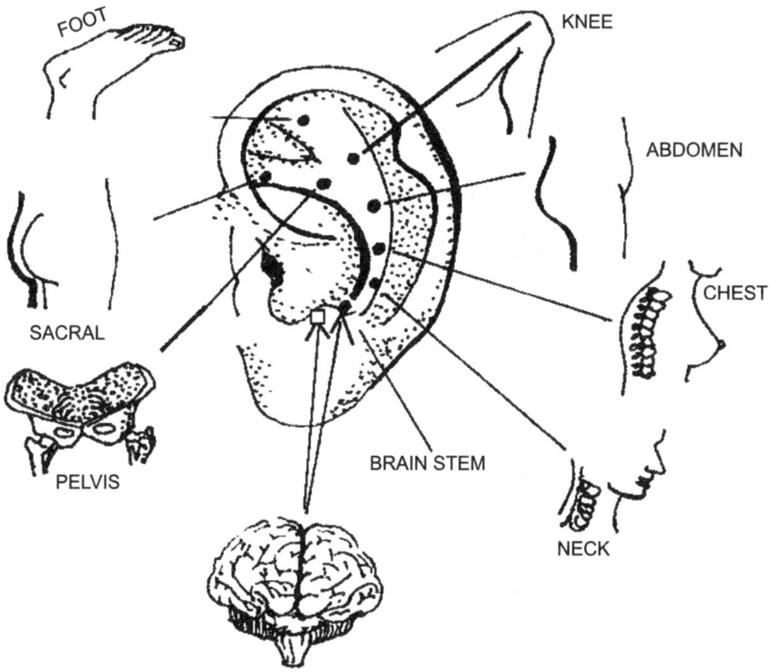

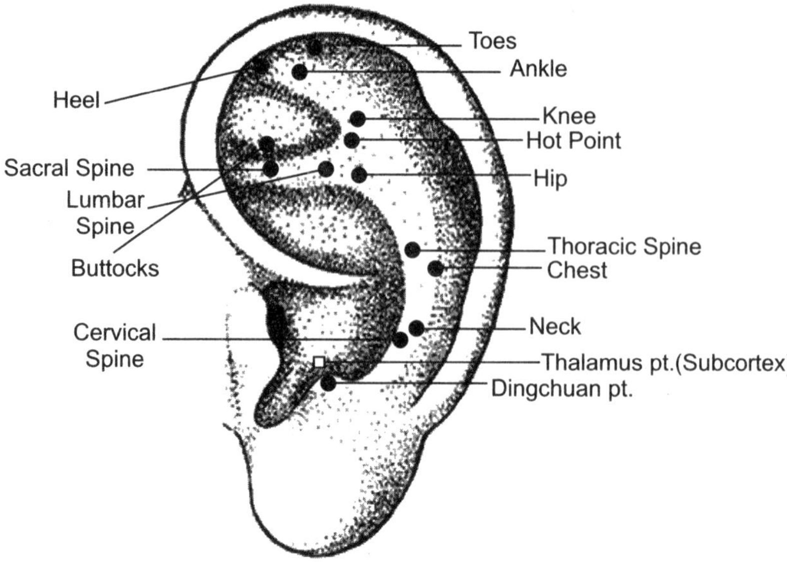

Outer side of anti-tragus

- Forehead, temporal and occiput area of the head.
- Headache, Insomnia, dizziness, sedation, pain relief.

Inner side of anti-tragus

- Subcortex area

LOWER HALF

- Pituitary hormone produced.

  Mental retardation, cerebral palsy, epilepsy, Parkinsonism, dream disturbed sleep, inflammation.

UPPER HALF

- Ovary and testis.
- For sterility, impotence, irregular menstruation.

Apex of anti-tragus

- Dingchuan point — A master point.

☞ For Asthma relief. Stimulating the point brings instant relief to asthma and lung-related problems.

Brain stem (Medulla)

👂 At the junction of anti-tragus and anti-helix.

☞ Headache, vertigo, relieving pain, allergy, stopping bleeding, easing mind, insomnia. Stabilises temperature, respiration, cardiac regulation.

Thalamus — A master point

👂 It is at the base of anti-tragus. It connects to cerebral cortex.

☞ It regulates overexcitement and restores tranquillity. It reduces chronic pain by activating inhibitory thalamus gate system. It regulates autonomic nerves used for all pain and brain-related problems.

Anti-Helix

This consists of the three parts:

1. The anti-helix stem.
2. Inferior crus of anti-helix.
3. Superior crus of anti-helix.

THE ANTI-HELIX STEM

This extends from brain stem to lower and inferior crus (as shown in the diagram).

The anti-helix stem represents the spinal column, the neck, chest and abdomen area.

The spinal column is represented by the ridge of anti-helix. Dividing the anti-helix into three parts from its starting point at anti-tragus junction to end point at inferior crus where it joins helix, the three groups of spinal vertebrae can be traced here. (see figure)

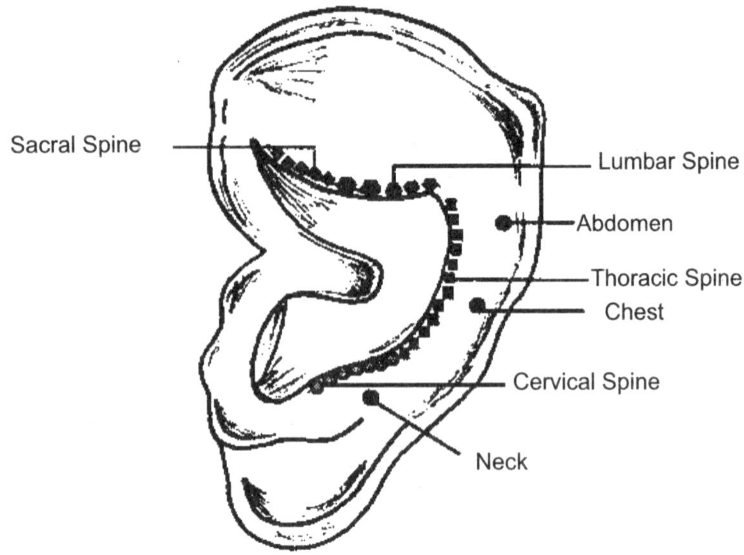

- **Neck area**
- Cervical spondylosis, sprain in neck, hyper and hypo thyroidism.
- **Chest area**
- Chest pain, intercostal neuralgia, upper back pain and shoulder pain.
- **Abdomen area**

  Pain in abdomen, menstrual pain, lower back pain, hernia and digestive problems.

INFERIOR CRUS OF ANTI-HELIX

It contains buttocks, pelvic girdle, lower end of lumbar vertebra and coccyx.

- **Pelvic girdle**
- At the junction of anti-helix stem and lower end of inferior crus is pelvic girdle.
- Relieves lower back pain, lumbago.

2. **Buttocks**

The entire inferior crus is represented by it.

Relieves pain due to constipation, piles, lumbago, etc.

SUPERIOR CRUS OF ANTI-HELIX

It contains toe, ankle, heel, lower leg and knee.

1. **Toe**

At the upper corner of superior crus of anti-helix, lateral and below apex of ear.

2. **Ankle**

Inner to the toe point at the upper border of superior crus of anti-helix.

3. **Heel**

Above ankle point close to helix border.

4. **Lower leg**

Along the length of superior crus of anti-helix from the junction to upper border. Stimulating these points relieves the pain and inflammation in the corresponding region.

5. **Knees**

At the junction of superior crus and inferior crus slightly on outer side.

Arthritis of knee joint, fracture, etc.

Hot point

At the junction of inferior crus of anti-helix and superior crus of anti-helix.

Relieves pain, relaxes vessel, used in acute lumbar pain. Brings relief during fever.

Scapha

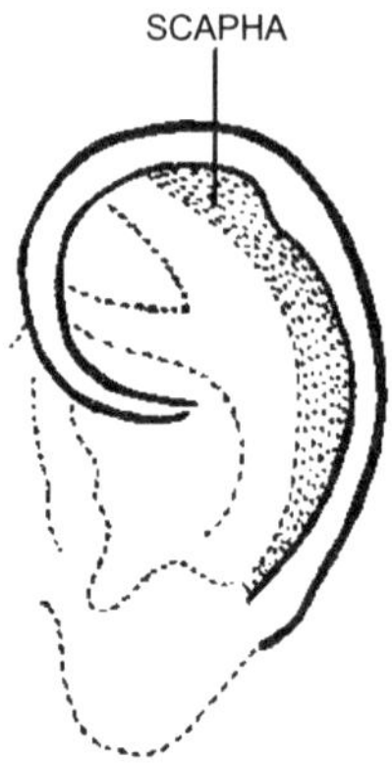

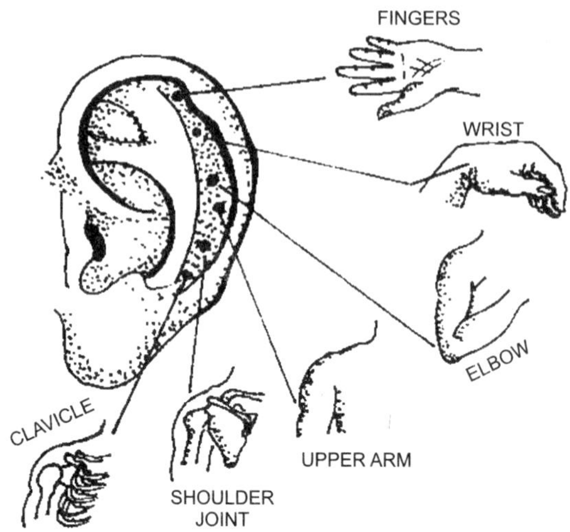

This represents the upper limb (i.e.) the hand.

In the scapha lie finger, wrist, lower arm, elbow, upper arm and shoulder in an upside down position as shown in the figure.

Clavicle

- In the starting point of anti-helix.
- ☞ Hemiplegia, numbness of hand, etc. Pain near clavicle, also useful to treat nephritis and appendix.

Shoulder Joint

- In level with supra-tragic notch.
- ☞ Dislocated shoulder, neck pain.

Elbow

- Between wrist and shoulder point.
- ☞ Elbow joint pain, tennis elbow.

Wrist

👂 At the point below Darwins tubercle.

☞ Wrist pain, immobility of wrist, arthritis.

Fingers

👂 Just above Darwins tubercle.

☞ Arthritis of fingers, problems in palm and fingers, sprain in fingers.

Helix

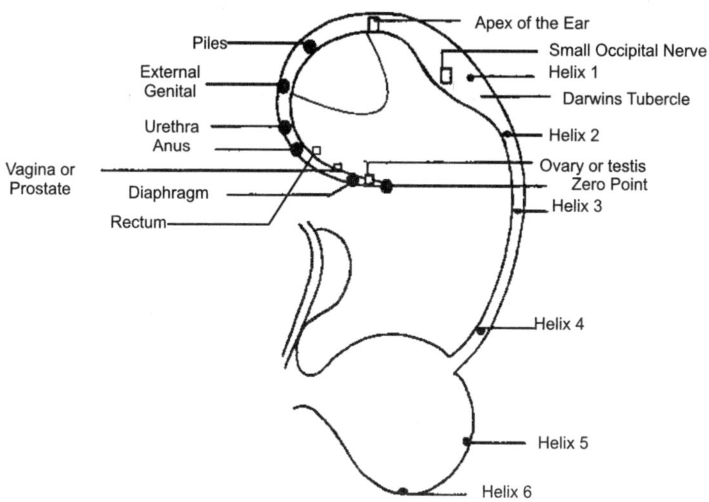

In the helix the important points are:

1. Apex of the ear – Point for allergy can be located by folding the ear.
2. Darwins tubercle – A prominent curve along the turning of the helix, opposite to the triangular fossa.
   (A very good homeostatic point for all organs in the body.)

3. The crus of helix – It is the tapering piece of helix as it enters the concave cavity. It represents anus, zero point and diaphragm.

Helix 1-6

- From the lower border of Darwins tubercule to lower border of lobe it is divided into 6 equal parts. Each is a trigger point corresponding to the outer surface of body.
- ☞ Used for acute pain, reducing heat in the body, acute tonsillitis.

Darwins tubercle (auricular tubercle)

- From ear apex the helix travels down and takes a turn opposite the triangular fossa. There the helix is slightly protruding and like a tubercle. This is called Darwins or auricular tubercle.
- ☞ Represents liver yang. Brings homoeostatis/balancing to zang fu organs, i.e. to all internal organs of the body.

  Turbulence in abdominal organs can be stabilised.

Apex of Ear — Allergy Point

- When the ear is folded vertically the topmost point represents the apex of the ear.
- ☞ Excess liver and heat decreases by piercing the point to bleed.

  All heat and excess conditions of the body can be treated from here. Used for hyperactivity, hypertension, irritable (getting angry soon), heat allergies, hyper pyrexia (high fever), acute tonsillitis conditions.

Zero point — A master point

- This is found at the end of crus of helix.
- ☞ Balancing point for energy and hormones. It is solar plexus point. It brings body to a homoeostatic state. A master point

to stabilise body's working used in all chronic problems. In case pain referrals are not located clearly, this point is first stimulated which will activate the ear.

Diaphragm

👂 On the helix crus just before the zero point close to external auditory meatus (the orifice).

☞ Hiccup, jaundice, spasms, blood and dermal disease, visceral (internal organ) haemorrhage.

Small occipital nerve

👂 On the medial surface of upper margin of auricular tubercle.

☞ It helps in sedation and relieving pain. Used for headache, vertigo, hemiplegia, numbness of hand, etc.

Openings of the body in the Helix

Helix holds number of openings of the body as it represents the outer cover of the body. They are:

Rectum

👂 On the end of helix near supra-tragic notch.

☞ Constipation, diarrhoea, prolapse of anus, incontinence of faeces, injury, fear caused by internal and external haemorrhoids.

Anus

👂 Found on the helix between lower segment of rectum and urethra.

☞ Constipation, itching in anus, prolapse, pain in lower back.

Vagina or prostate

👂 At the root of upper ear as the crus of helix enters the conchae in the inner side.

☞ Relieves prostate enlargement, vaginal itching, infection, etc.

Ovary or testis

- Found close to zero point in the inner fold of crus of helix.
- ☞ Treats sexual dysfunctions, impotence, frigidity, cystitis of ovary, etc.

Urethra

- At the part of helix in level with urinary bladder on the lower border of inferior crus of helix.
- ☞ Retention of urine, frequency and urgency in urine passing.

External genital organs

- Above urethra close to inferior crus of helix in level with its upper border.
- ☞ Impotence, eczema, skin eruption near external genital organ.

Haemorrhoid spot

- Upper part of helix at the upper border of superior crus of helix.
- ☞ Treats piles, bleeding, itching and prolapse of anus.

The Triangular Deltoid Fossa

Encircled by inferior crus of anti-helix and superior crus of anti-helix this triangular depression lies on the upper end of the ear. It contains some important therapeutic points:

1. Ear shenmen point	A very important point for treatment.
2. Blood pressure lowering point	At the top of the triangle.
3. Sympathetic nerve point	At the lower end of the triangle.
4. Sciatic nerve point	At the mid-lower base of the triangle.

5. Constipation point	At the lower base of the triangle close to sciatic nerve point.
6. Uterus point/ Prostate	Mid-point of the triangle along the base close to helix.

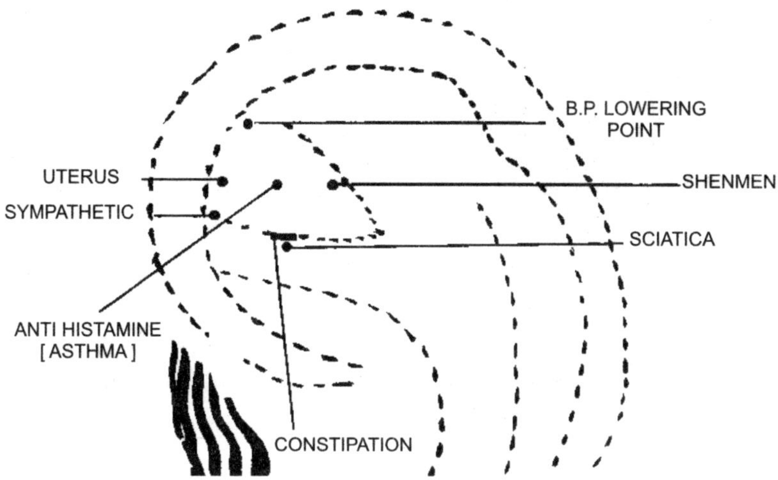

Shenmen — A master point

- It is found superior and central to curving tip of triangular fossa.

- Stimulating this point produces strong sedative and analgesic effect. Tranquillises mind and allows connection to one's spirit, alleviates stress, pain, tension, anxiety, depression, insomnia, restlessness, excessive sensitivity.

  Most commonly used point, a pallative in most of the disorders. Reduces fever, inflammatory diseases, epilepsy, high blood pressure, drives off heat, counteracts poison.

Sciatica Nerve Point

- At the mid-point on the base of the triangle.

- Relieves greatly sciatica pain.

Constipation point

- This coincides with sciatic nerve.
- ☞ Used for piles and constipation.

Sympathetic nerve point — A master point

- This is found at the lower end of triangular fossa, close to helix in the inferior crus of anti-helix.
- ☞ Improves various involuntary actions of the body.

  Used to treat spasmodic pain and spasms. Angina pectoris, renal colic, abdominal pain, improves circulation, disease of digestive and circulatory system. Stress relief, dysmenorrhea (painful menstruation). Uretory colloid, hyperhydrosis (increased sweating) and night sweat. This point is also used for acupuncture in throat and abdominal operation.

Uterus/Prostate point

- Close to base of triangular fossa as shown in figure.
- ☞ Uterus-related problems. Irregular menstruation, painful periods, excessive bleeding, impotence, nocturnal emission, prostate, etc.

Point of lowering blood pressure

- This is found in the upper corner of triangular fossa close to superior crus of anti-helix.
- ☞ Lowers the blood pressure. Used for high blood pressure and related cardiac problems.

Asthma point — Anti-histamine point

- This is found 0.2 mm lateral and lower to uterus point.
- ☞ This is yet another point for treating asthma. Treats asthma attacks effectively.

Tragus

The flap crossing the ear orifice attached to the face is tragus. It mainly represents nose and a part of pharynx and larynx. And it also has important points like hunger point, adrenal point, etc.

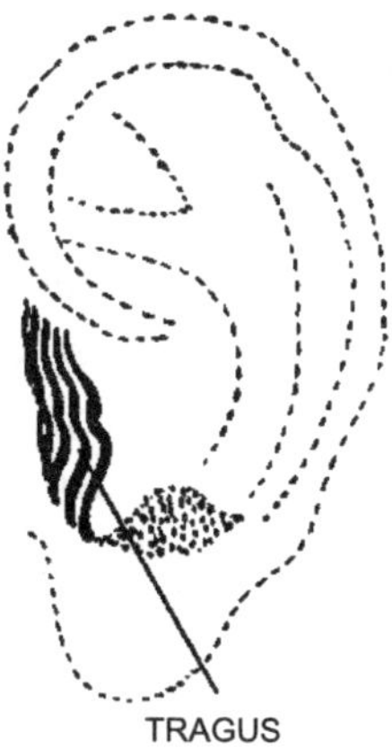

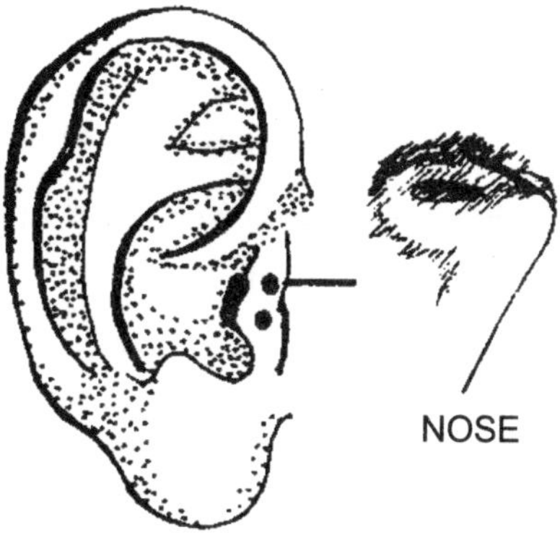

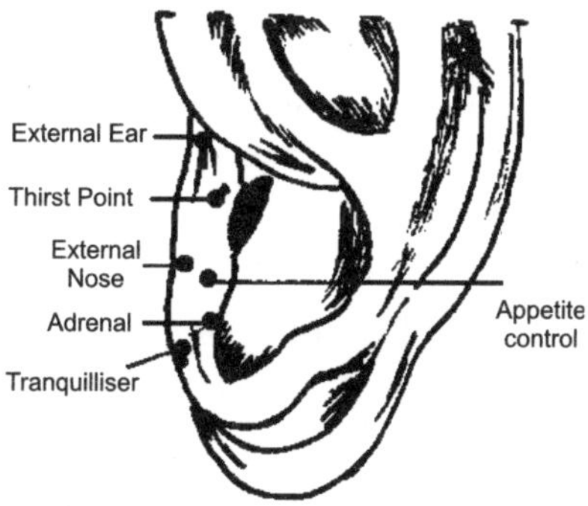

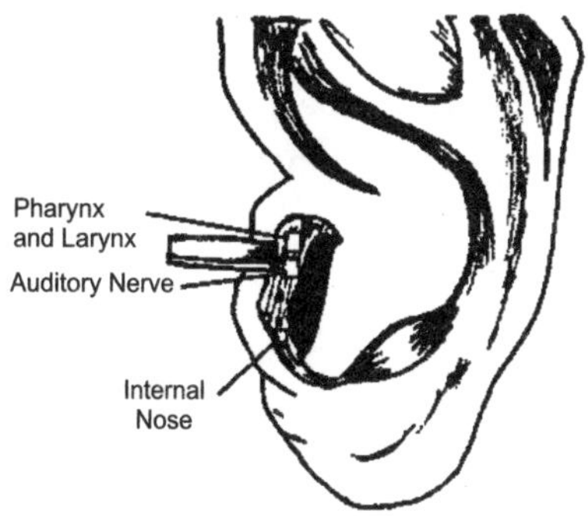

External nose

- In the centre of the lateral side close to face.

☞ Cold, rhinitis, nose block.

Pharynx and Larynx

- In the inside of tragus on the upper half.

☞ Pharyngitis, laryngitis, tonsillitis.

Internal nose

👂 In the inside of tragus on the lower half.

☞ Cold, sinusitis, growth inside nose, deviation of the bone, difficulty in breathing.

Adrenal point — A Master point

👂 At the lower end of tragus on the border. This is in the apex of the intra-tragic notch.

☞ Regulates adernal gland and cortical hormone.

Eliminates inflammation, swelling, anti-allergy, rheumatism, anti-infection, does arterio vaso dilation and vaso constriction and stops bleeding, hypertension, haemorrhage, reduces high fever, low grade fever, cough, soothes asthma, dermal disease.

Hunger point (appetite control)

👂 It is in the middle of tragus just behind the orifice.

☞ Pressing the point repeatedly before mealtime decreases the appetite considerably.

Thirst Point

👂 Found directly above appetite control point.

☞ Diminishes excessive thirst.

Tranquilliser point.

👂 Close to adrenal point but on lateral side close to face. Brings sedation effect, brings overall relaxation.

☞ Reduces high blood pressure and chronic stress. Also referred as relaxation point.

Cavum Conchae (Inter-tragic Notch and Supra-tragic Notch)

All the internal soft organs lie in the concave space inside, which is divided into two parts by the crus of helix — upper cymba conchae where the lower abdominal parts lie and lower cavum conchae in which the upper abdominal parts lie.

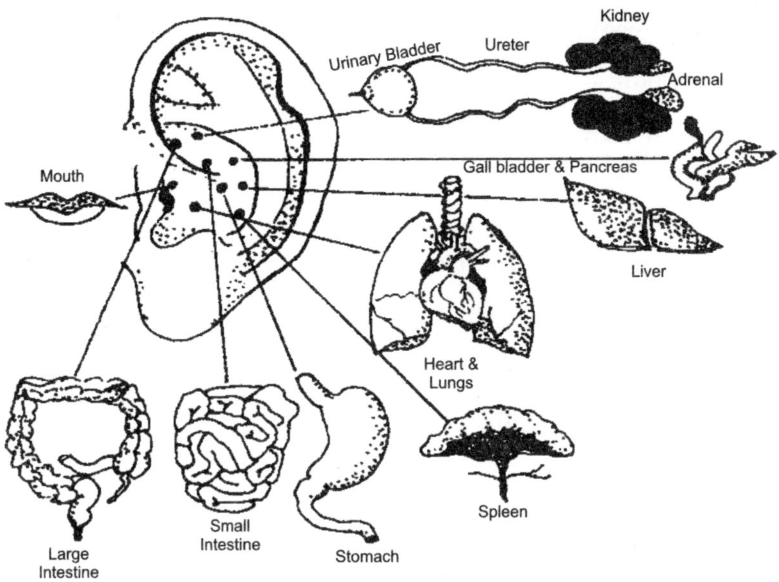

The inter-tragic notch and supra-tragic notch are two depressions on either side of cavum conchae. The inter-tragic notch is towards the lobe. It represents mainly the sub-cortical region of the brain. The supra-tragic notch is towards the orifice of the ear facing the tragus. It represents mainly the nose, both the external and internal aspects.

Cavum Conchae

Represents the parts above diaphragm, mainly heart and lungs.

Heart

- It is in the deepest part of cavum conchae in the centre in between the two lungs.
- ☞ Treating heart point helps in relieving circulatory problems and mental problems as heart energy controls mind (refer heart functional notes).

Lung

- Lying horizontally on either side of heart are the two lungs. The one lying on lower side represents lung of the same side.

  The one lying on the upper side of heart represents lung of the opposite side (the left lung is smaller having 2 lobes, the right lung has 3 lobes).
- ☞ Treating lung point helps all respiratory problems and the skin problems as lung energy guards the skin layer.

  Lung point also extensively used to treat addictions such as smoking and other substance addictions like tobacco chewing, *gutka,* etc.

Trachea

- Between mouth point and heart point.
- ☞ Treats cough and bronchitis.

Mouth, Oesophagus, Cardiac orifice and Part of stomach

They lie hugging the crus of helix.

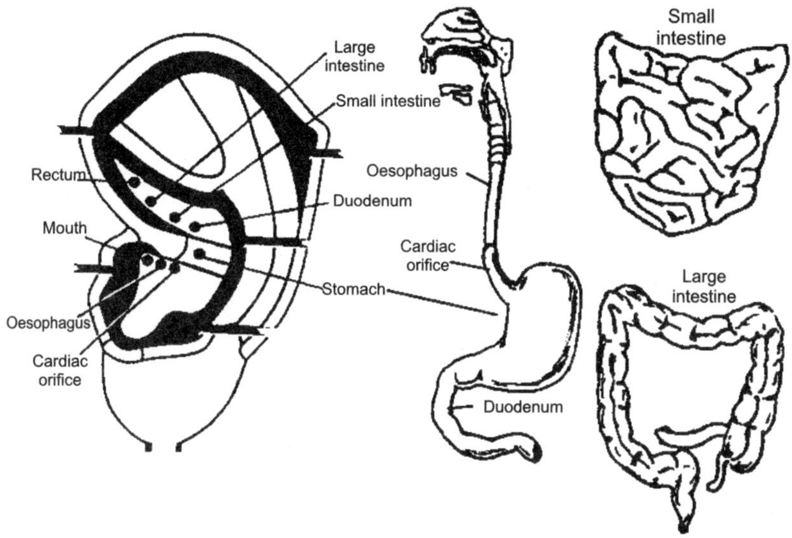

Alimentry canal

Mouth

- It lies close to orifice below the crus of helix.
- ☞ The area around the mouth point is also extensively used as another hunger point. It is used for treating obesity. It also treats problems related to mouth like gum problem, salivary gland infection, chewing problem, facial paralysis, etc.

Oesophagus

- Extending from mouth in the lower side of crus of helix for a distance of one finger width is oesophagus.
- ☞ The oesophagus area treats difficulty of swallowing, carcinoma, tumor in the tube, etc. The needling should be done towards alimentary canal. Also treats hiatus hernia when stomach portion goes inside oesophagus.

Cardiac Orifice

- This lies next to oesophagus, below zero point.
- ☞ It is the opening of the oesophagus into the stomach. Treats the blockage of this orifice, swallowing problems, nausea, vomiting. A condition ankylosing hernia is treated (when oesophagus resembles a rat tail).

Stomach

- Stomach lies exactly hugging the crus of helix, part of it in cavum conchae and part of it in cymba conchae.
- ☞ Treats digestive problems of stomach as well as gastric ulcer, acidity.

Spleen

- This is found below stomach along conchae wall. This point is more prominently traced in left ear as spleen is anatomically on the left side.
- ☞ It treats digestive, immunity and dermal problems. It is also used for obesity control, hernia, gas problem and anaemia.

Vagus nerve

- It is found at the apex of trachea point below mouth, the nerve however spreads throughout conchae.
- ☞ It affects the parasympathetic nervous system and controls most of thoracic and abdominal organs. It relieves heart palpitation, anxiety, digestive disturbance like diarrhoea, indigestion.

The wall of conchae along anti-tragus

This represents brain stem, brain, sub-cortex and thalamus.

- ☞ It treats neurological problems.

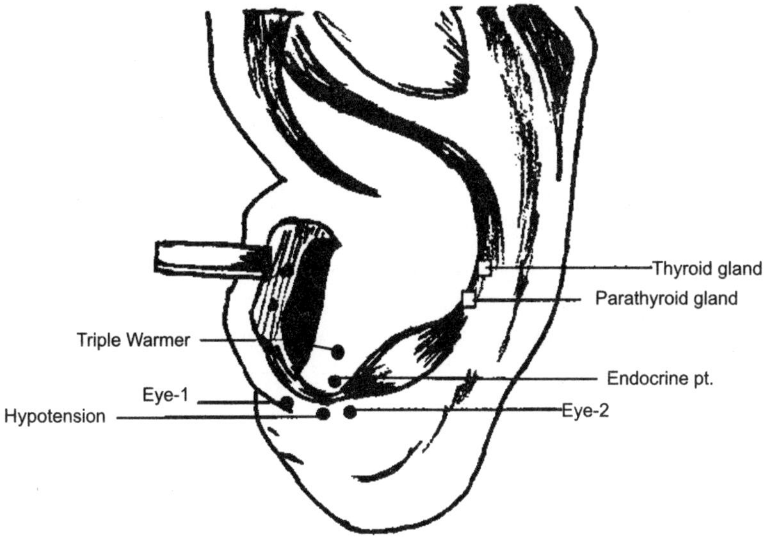

Thyroid gland

- It is found in the inner wall of conchae, above brain stem, behind anti-helix starting point.
- ☞ It treats hypo and hyperthyroidism which in turn affects the metabolism of the body.

Parathyroid gland

- Below thyroid gland is the parathyroid gland.
- ☞ It affects calcium metabolism. It helps in relieving muscle cramps and muscle spasm.

Inter-tragic notch

- The inner side of the notch contains two important points. Endocrine point containing pituitary body and triple warmer point.

  The outer side of the notch contains eye 1 and eye 2 and hypotension point between them.

Endocrine point — It is a master point

- It is found lodged in the deeper lowest portion of the intertragic notch.

- ☞ It holds the pituitary body which controls the other endocrine glands in the body. It helps in secreting hormones at proper homoeostatic level either rising or lowering glandular secretions. Activates pituitary gland below brain which is the master gland controlling the other glands. Relieves rheumatism, urinogenital disorders, dermal disease, disorders in the gastrointestinal tract and re-occurring fevers like malaria.

Triple warmer

- Found above the endocrine point, on the upper part of the intertragic notch.

- ☞ It maintains the proper homeostatic level in the trunk cavity which houses all the organs.

  Helps in problems like hypertension, stopping bleeding, etc. Anti-allergic and anti-inflammatory.

Eye 1 and Eye 2

- It lies on either side of inter-tragic notch.

- ☞ Treats glaucoma, myopia, hordeolum, poor eyesight.

Hypotension

- Found at the centre of inter-tragic notch on the outer side.

- ☞ Elevates abnormally low blood pressure.

Cymba Conchae

In the upper concave cavity above the crus of helix lies the cymba conchae.

1. In the cymba conchae lie rest of the alimentary canal, the kidney, urinary bladder, urethra and rest of the lower abdominal portion.

2. The crus of helix on the cymba conchae side has part of the stomach, duodenum, small intestine, appendix, large intestine and rectum (fig. shown in alimentary canal dig).
3. The kidney, ureter, urinary bladder and prostate lie along the upper border of cavum conchae.

   Above the small intestine lies the kidney.

   Above large intestine lie the ureter and urinary bladder.
4. The pancreas, gall bladder, liver, spleen, lie along the outer edge of cymba conchae in the inner border of anti-helix as shown in figure.

   (The pancreas can be located in the left ear while the gall bladder in the right ear.)
5. On the inner wall close to stomach is liver.

   Pancreas lies above duodenum next to liver in the left ear.

   Gall bladder lies above duodenum next to liver in the right ear.

   Ascites point lies between kidney and small intestine.

   It can be used for the treatment of oedema or swelling.

   This is also termed as alcoholic point. Assists in treatment of alchoholism, relieves hangovers.

The spleen lies below the liver on the conchae wall.

Liver

- It lies in the diaphragm line (the crus of helix) just behind stomach, a part of it spilling on the conchae wall.

  (Liver is a huge organ weighing 1.5 kg.) (Liver points are also found as liver yang in the auricular tubercle while liver excess can be corrected at the apex of the ear.)

☞ Stimulating the point helps in improving digestion, working of muscles and tendons, (decreases muscular pain).

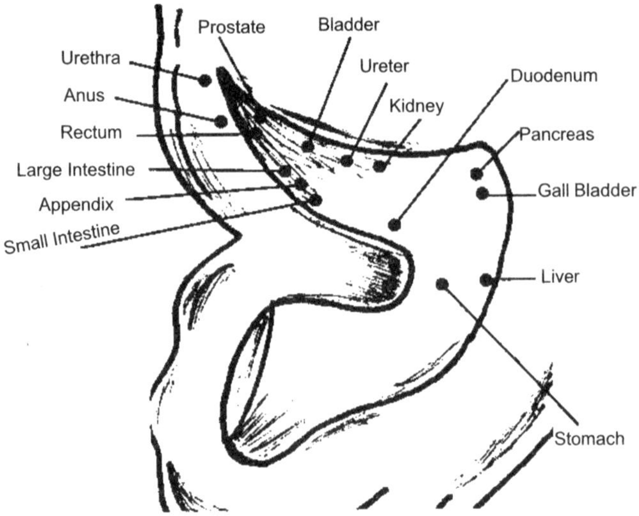

The homoeostatic (balance) operation of liver improves eyesight, helps in infertility, impotence and menstruation problems.

Liver excess can be controlled at ear apex by pricking the point to bleed and bring down heat in the liver.

Gall bladder

In the right ear

- It lies above liver in the upper part of cavum conchae, bove the duodenum point.

- Gall bladder stores the bile. Stimulating the point helps in digestion, clears gall bladder stones, diseases of bile duct.

  As its meridian energy runs over the head, encircles ear and comes down along lateral aspect of leg close to sciatic nerve, a treatment in this helps headache (migraine), deafness, sciatica and severe leg pain and cramps [see gall bladder notes]. Also helps to clear liver energy stagnation.

Pancreas

In the left ear

- It lies above liver point in the left ear.

☞ Helps in metabolic process, rejuvenating pancreas and **improves diabetic condition admirably**. Also helps in pancreatitis, migraine.

The kidney, ureter, urinary bladder, urethra (opening) all lie in a row:

Kidney	:	Above small intestine.
Ureter	:	Above appendix.
Urinary bladder	:	Above large intestine.
Urethra	:	Above anus in the helix.

Kidney

- This lies above small intestine in the cavum conchae just above where the anti-helix takes a turn.

☞ Kidney is an organ controlling multi-activities in the body. Stimulating the point helps in correcting

– Renal failure

As kidney governs bone and cartilage it helps:

– Arthritis

– Spondylosis

As kidney energy opens to ears it helps:

– Deafness, tinnitus (ringing in ears)

As kidney governs genital organs it helps:

– Sterility (oligospermia, azospermia)

– Development of ovary and uterus

– Menstruation problems

– It also improves teeth and hair.

– It removes excess fire from body.

– This helps in controlling burning urine.

– Bleeding gums, epilepsy

Kidney helps in increasing life (see kidney energy functional notes).

Adrenal glands

👂 This lies above kidney in the cavum conchae in the turning of anti-helix (this is a second stimulating point of adrenal, another lies in tragus)

☞ Stimulating the point brings in improving function of adrenal gland (see notes on adrenal in tragus notes).

Ureter

👂 It lies next to kidney above appendix point and further.

☞ Useful to treat blockage of ureter by stone, colic pain, etc.

Urinary bladder

👂 It lies above large intestine in the lower border of inferior anti-helix crus.

☞ Helps in clearing bladder-related problems:

- Backache
- Sciatica
- Cyst in bladder
- Retention of urine, incontinence of urine
- Prostatis and nephritis are also treated at this point (see urinary bladder notes).

Urethra

👂 It lies on the helix below inferior crus of anti-helix.

☞ Treats frequent urgent painful urination, retention of urine, burning urine, itching around urethra.

Stomach

- The stomach lies in the crus of helix party in cavum conchae and partly in cymba conchae.
- Hyperacidity, gastric ulcer, lack of appetite, vomiting and nausea.

Duodenum

- Lies next to stomach on the opposite side of cardiac orifice.
- Duodenal ulcer, spasm in stomach due to duodenal blockage.

Small intestine

- Next to duodenum, on the upper part of crus of helix opposite to oesophagus.
- Digestive problems, lack of absorption, diarrhoea, indigestion, abdominal distention, intestinal tuberculosis.

  As it is connected to heart by meridian it helps to treat heart troubles such as palpitation, short of breath.

Appendix

- This lies in the junction between small intestine and large intestine.
- During inflammation of appendix there is pain here, appendicitis.

Large Intestine

- Next to small intestine in the anterior 1/3rd of upper part of crus of helix.
- Diarrhoea, constipation, ulcer in the large intestine, incontinence of faeces, colitis, irritable bowel syndrome. As large intestine is connected to lung by meridian it also treats respiratory disorders.

Rectum

- Lower portion of large intestine where it meets helix.
- ☞ Treats piles, haemorrhoids, rectum prolapse.

Anus

- On the helix just next to rectum.
- ☞ Treats piles, haemorrhoids, anal fissure.

The Back of the Ear

The yang side or the posterior side of the ear is not routinely used. However body representation on yang side can be used when cure effect is not appreciable by using the yin side alone. Also for certain ailments like back pain, sciatica, blood pressure and for some neurological problems back of the ear shows good cure effect.

Precautions using the yang side:

1. Don't use simultaneously the yin and yang side of the auricle.
2. Care should be taken in needle penetration as the cartilage is more pronounced in the yang side and deeper penetration can lead to infection.

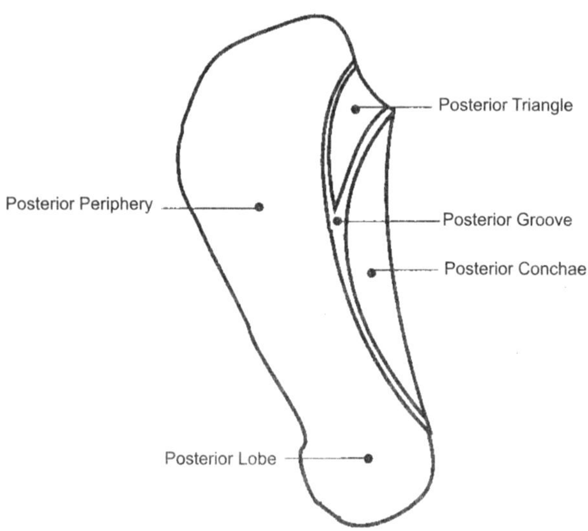

Organs of the Body

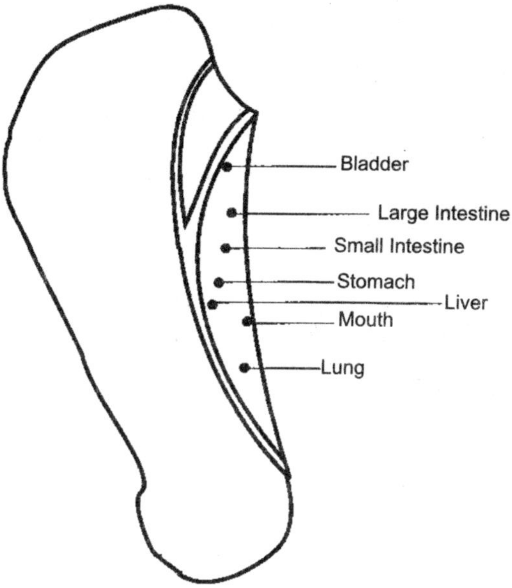

Ear Points for Corresponding Body Area

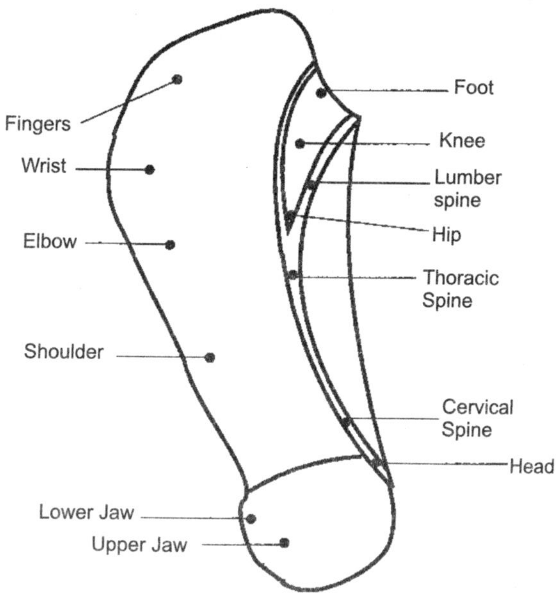

Posterior Auricular Zones for Nervous System

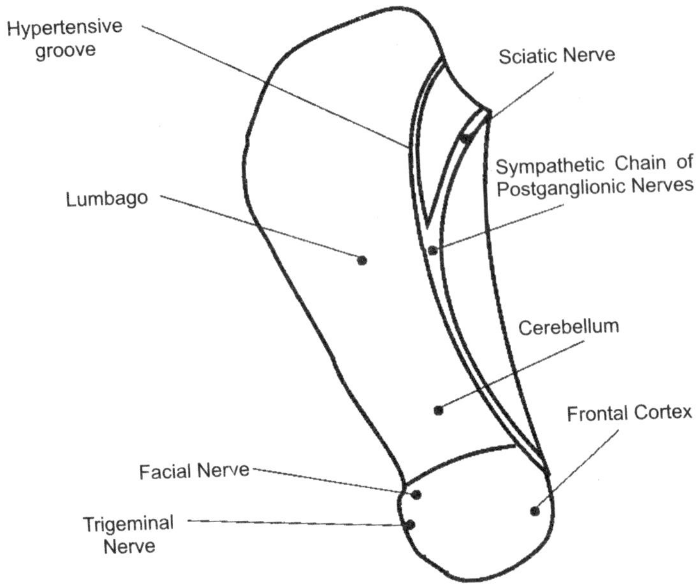

3

Important Therapeutic Points

Master Points

THE ear has many important therapeutic points bringing in effective chemical and metabolic changes in the body mechanism and accelerating cure. These points are like broad spectrum medicines used for a vast variety of health disorders. The primary and secondary master points are listed here for quick reference.

The Primary Master Points

1. Shenmen
2. Point zero
3. Thalamus point
4. Endocrine point
5. Sympathetic (Autonomic nerve point)
6. Adrenal point
7. Allergy point
8. Dingchuan point (asthma point)

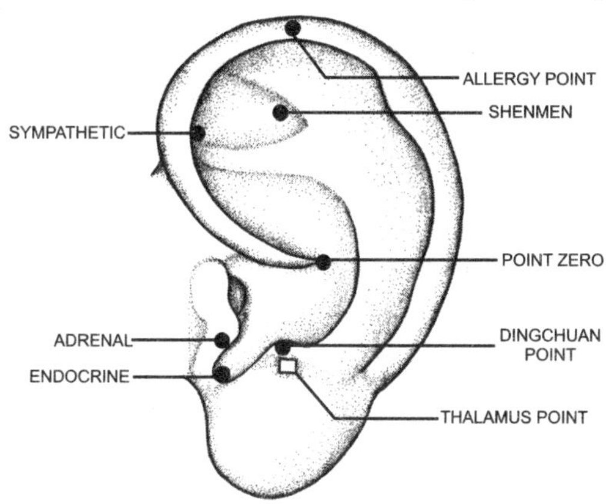

Points shown in figure, function and detailed description.

1. **Shenmen point :** It is the best sedative and analgesic point in the ear. It is combined with other points for treatment. It has broad spectrum action like antibiotic.

2. **Zero point** : This point is found at the end of crus of helix. Right in the centre of the ear as shown in the figure. It acts on the solar plexus through the vagus nerve.

   It is also used as the pain referral point. The point is generally painful on all the patients. Stimulating this point in the beginning will bring out to the surface the other sensitive points in the ear for treatment.

3. **Hypothalamus point :** It is at the base of anti-tragus. It is an important glandular control point found anatomically below brain. Stimulating this point fetches good results in paralysis, spasms, arthritis, etc. and helps in controlling pain.

4. **Endocrine point :** This is useful for all endocrine disorders and also used to help in drug withdrawal symptoms when the patient is coming out of heavy drugs like steroids, cortisones, etc. It acts as master of endocrine gland, stimulating other endocrine glands to action.

   It is also referred to as internal secretion point.

5. **Sympathetic nerve point :** It is in the end of deltoid fossa in the lower portion close to the inferior crus of the helix. It helps in improvement of autonomic nervous system and helps digestive, circulatory, respiratory systems.

6. **Adrenal point :** At the lower end of the tragus above the notch. It acts as emergency point boosting the energy level of the body to tide over the crisis.

7. **Allergy point** : Found at the internal side of the apex of the ear. It leads to the reduction of inflammation and heat reactions during allergies, arthritis and asthma.

Helps in removing the toxins. At times pricking it to bleed helps in bringing down heat.

8. **Dingchuan point :** It is a very effective point for relieving asthma. It is found at the tip of anti-tragus at the sub-cortex of the brain.

Secondary Master Points

The secondary master points are:

1. Master cerebral
2. Master sensorial
3. Thyroid point
4. Tranquilliser point
5. Root of helix
6. Darwins tubercle
7. Point for lowering blood pressure
8. Sciatic nerve point
9. Oedema or ascites point
10. Appetite control
11. Muscle Relaxation point
12. Pancreas point
13. Hot point
14. The line of sound
15. Constipation point
16. Urticaria point.

1. **Master cerebral :** It is found in the lobe below the teeth point, at the side where the ear meets the face. It represents the pre-frontal lobe of the brain which is involved in decision-making. Stimulation of this point relieves excess worry, nervous anxiety, pessimistic thinking and other psychosomatic problems.

2. **Master sensorial :** It coincides with the eye point in the middle of the lobe. It controls the sensory cortex area of the brain. It helps to control excessive sensitivity in the body, thus relieving a burning tingling sensation in the body, ringing in ears, blurred vision, etc.

3. **Thyroid point :** It is found in the inner conchae wall above sub-cortex region. Helps in regulating thyroid function both in hypo- and hyperthyroidism.

4. **Tranquilliser point** : Found in tragus as it joins the face. It brings in general relaxation. It stimulates the pineal gland

of the brain bringing in relaxation and sleep. It relieves chronic stress and also helps in hypertension reduction.

Secondary Master Points

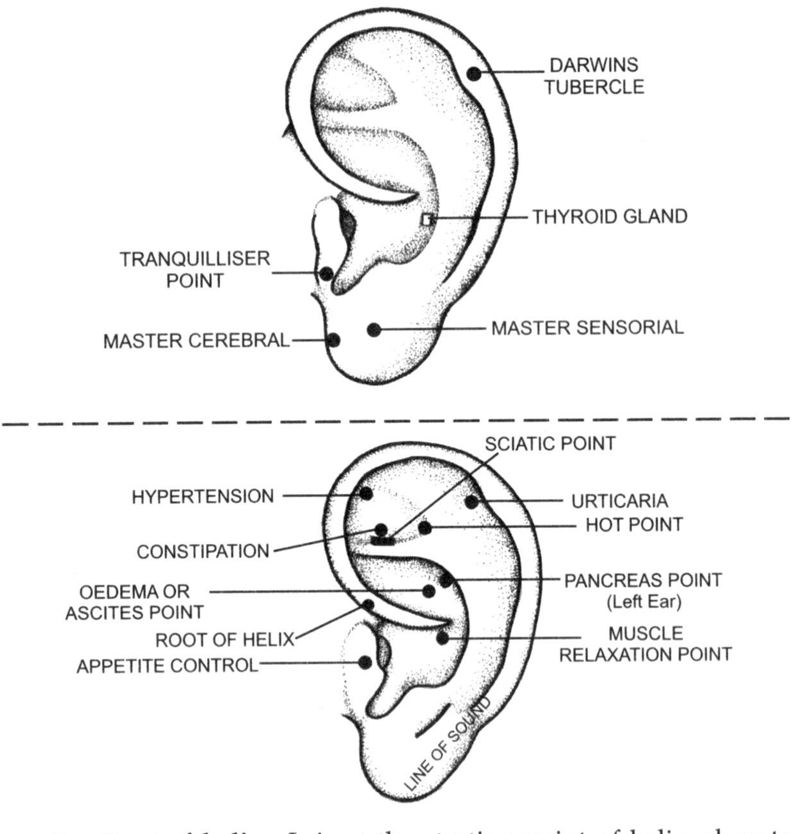

5. **Root of helix :** It is at the starting point of helix, close to tragus. It is attached to trigeminal nerve. Tenderness at this point denotes anxiety in the patient or emotional disturbance.

   The zero point combined with root of helix point takes care of the normalisation of the organs, both hypo- and hyperactivity.

6. **Darwins tubercle :** It is also called earth energy point. It separates the trigeminal and sympathetic cervical plexus.

It acts as a good balancing point and useful in correcting internal organ disorders.

7. **Point of lowering blood pressure :** In the deltoid fossa, in the upper portion of the triangle. Also the groove of the back of the ear is effective for lowering the blood pressure. (The groove starts in the yang side behind blood pressure point.)
8. **Sciatic nerve point :** The anterior half of the inferior crus of anti-helix represents the sciatic nerve area.
9. **Oedema/Ascites point :** It is in the cymba conchae, in the middle between small intestine and kidney. It helps in bringing down swelling in the body.
10. **Appetite control :** In the lower and inner side of tragus close to the cheek. Pressing this point half an hour before the meals brings down the appetite.
11. **Muscle relaxation point :** In the cavum conchae between spleen and the lungs. It helps in muscle relaxation.
12. **Pancreas point :** In the cymba conchae in the outer rim, above the ridge of crus of helix. It is found only in the left ear. In the right ear the same position is taken by gall bladder.
13. **Hot point :** It is at the apex of deltoid fossa further to shenmen. It is useful for bringing down the temperature during fever.
14. **The line of sound :** In the scapha the portion close to anti-tragus leading to the lobe is known as the line of sound and is useful for treating deafness, tinnitus, vertigo and Meneiere's diseases.
15. **Constipation point :** It is found in the lower side of the triangular deltoid fossa, lying close to hip joint area.
16. **Urticaria point :** It is found opposite Darwins tubercle in the scapha region. It helps in allergy and itching of the skin.

Endocrine Glands

Endocrine glands, the ductless glands are very important for our general well-being. They secrete chemical hormones in small quantities which mix up with our system and help in various vital functions of the body.

In all there are seven important endocrine glands; they are:

1. Pineal
2. Pituitary (anterior pituitary, posterior pituitary)
3. Thyroid and parathyroid
4. Thymus
5. Adrenal
6. Pancreas
7. Gonads (ovary and testis)

The location, hormones secreted by them and their functions are as follows:

1. Pineal

- Found at the lowermost part of tragus.
- Situated above mid-brain and below cerebral cortex.
- Release melatonin hormone.
- Regulates sleep patterns, used in insomnia, jet lag, depression, etc.

2. Pituitary

- There are two pituitary bodies: anterior pituitary and posterior pituitary.

Anterior pituitary

- Found in the inter-tragic notch in the lowermost portion.
- Situated in the mid-brain below hypothalamus.

- This is the master endocrine gland.
- It controls the release of hormones from all other endocrine glands.
- It releases varied hormones such as ACTH, TSH, FSH, LH, endorphins and growth hormones.
- Helps in treating reproductive disorders, allergies, arthritis, diseases of circulatory, digestive system, skin diseases, etc. It also triggers other endocrine glands to function. Hence it is called master endocrine point or internal secretions.

Endocrine Glands

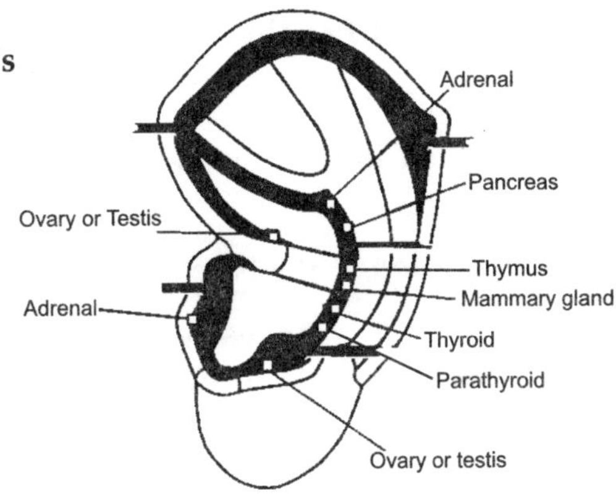

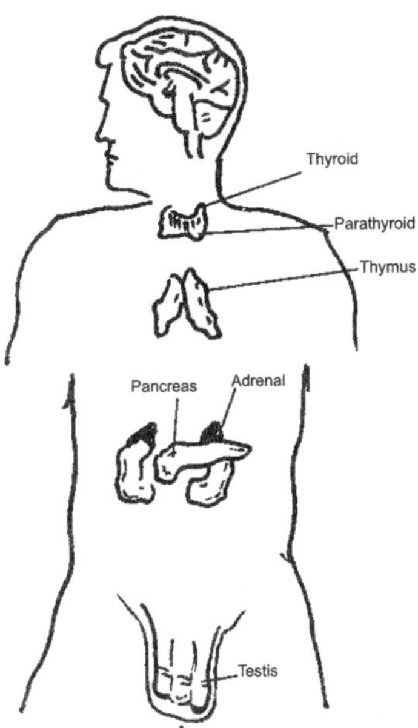

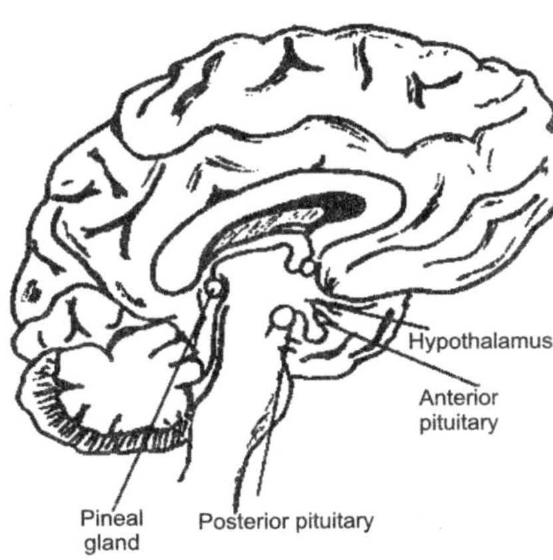

Note: ACTH - Adrenocorticotropic hormone. TSH - Thyroid stimulating harmone. FSH - Follicle stimulating harmone. LH - Lutcinizing harmone. ADH - Anti diuretic harmone.

Posterior pituitary

- Found above anterior pituitary along the tragus side.
- Situated below hypothalamus.
- Secretes ADH and oxytocin hormones.
- ADH is antidiuretic hormone which controls thirst, internal water regulation and salt metabolism.
- Oxytocin hormone helps in uterine contraction in child birth.

3. Thyroid and Parathyroid

(i) Thyroid

- Found in the inner wall of anti-helix in cavum conchae as shown.
- Situated at the base of the throat.
- Thyroid secretes thyroxin — It helps in cellular metabolism concerned with glucose reduction and iron deficiency (Thyrotropin (TSH)) is also secreted by anterior pituitary which aids the release of thyroxin.

(ii) Parathyroid

- Lies next to thyroid.
- Releases parathormone in the blood, helps in maintaining calcium level in blood. It in turn affects nervous system excitability.

4. Thymus

- Found in the inner wall of anti-helix in cymba conchae as shown
- Situated behind the sternum in the chest.
- Helps in differentiation of white blood cells to active immune cells.
- Treates cold, flu, allergies, cancer, HIV, Aids.

5. Adrenal

- There are two adrenal points. One found in the inner wall of anti-helix in cymba conchae where the ear takes a turn, another at the lower end of the tragus.
- It is situated at the top of each kidney.
- Secretes adrenalin and cortisol hormone.
- Adrenalin hormone activates sympathetic nerves and helps in regulating the working of internal organs. Cortisol hormone helps in relief of stress-related problems.

  (In anterior pituitary ACTH is secreted which helps the functioning of main adrenal gland.)

6. Pancreas

- Found above duodenum in the left ear at cymba conchae.
- Situated next to stomach.
- Releases the hormone insulin.
- Helps in transportation of glucose (sugar) from the blood to the cells and converting it into glycogen (energy).

7. Gonads : Sex Glands (Ovary and Testis)

- The trigger points of the sex glands are found near the pituitary body at the sub-cortex region. They release gonadal hormones FSH and LH which activate the ovaries and testes to secrete the sex hormones. (Ovaries are situated in pelvic cavity. Testes in men are situated outside pelvic cavity.) They are found in the under side of the crus of helix close to zero point anatomically.
- Ovaries release progesterone and estrogen.
- Testes release testosterone.
- The anterior pituitary releases gonadal hormones FSH and, LH (which activate ovary and testes functioning).
- Relieves sexual dysfunction, impotence, irregular menstruation, etc.

4

The Chinese Functional Meridian Points

THE Chinese with their long-standing wisdom acquired the knowledge of how each of the vital organs of the body operates functionally and is in charge of the various workings in the body.

The information given here is the one used in classical acupuncture which is based on the energy meridians of the body, or in short how the energy of the different organs operates in the body.

On stimulation the following organ points in the ear:

Heart

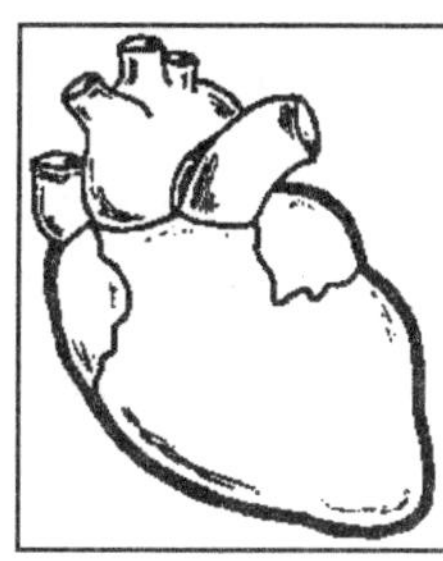

Regulates	:	Circulation of blood
Rules	:	Mental activity
Governs	:	Sweat
Opens	:	In tongue
Holds	:	Spirit
Represents	:	Fire element

Stimulating this point helps:

(i) To calm heart and mind.

(ii) Eliminate heat of heart.

(iii) Treats diseases of cardiaovascular system, heart trouble, palpitation, shortness of breath.

(iv) Treats mental diseases

(a) Anxiety, (b) Depression, (c) Amnesia

(v) Excess sweating — as heart controls sweat

(vi) As heart energy passes through throat and opens in the tongue, it treats: (a) Pharyngitis, (b) Hoarseness, (c) Pain in tongue, (d) Glossitis and (e) Stomatitis.

Lungs

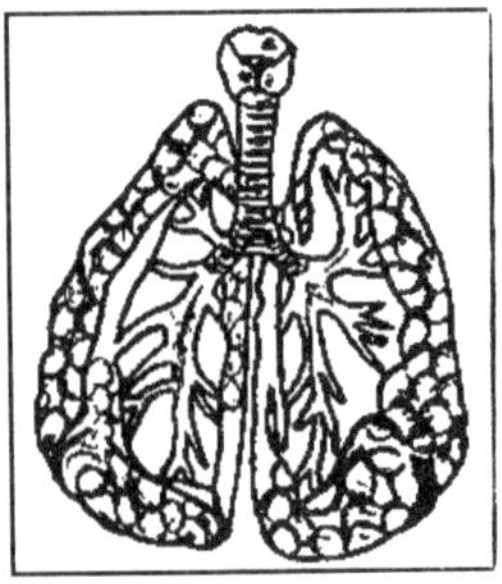

Regulates	:	Respiration
Rules	:	Skin and body hair
Governs	:	Mucus
Opens	:	To nose
Holds	:	'Qi' or *praana*
Represents	:	Metal element

Stimulating this point helps:

(i) Diseases of respiratory system: (a) Common cold, (b) Cold sweat, (c) Pulmonary tuberculosis, (d) Cough, (e) Asthma, (f) Sore throat, and (g) Hoarseness.

(ii) Improves circulation of blood and energy.

(iii) Helps in various dermal diseases.

(iv) Lung energy is connected to large intestine through meridian. Hence helps in colon disorders.

(v) This point is used widely in ear acupuncture anaesthesia as it immediately brings analgesis on the surface of the skin for incision.

Liver

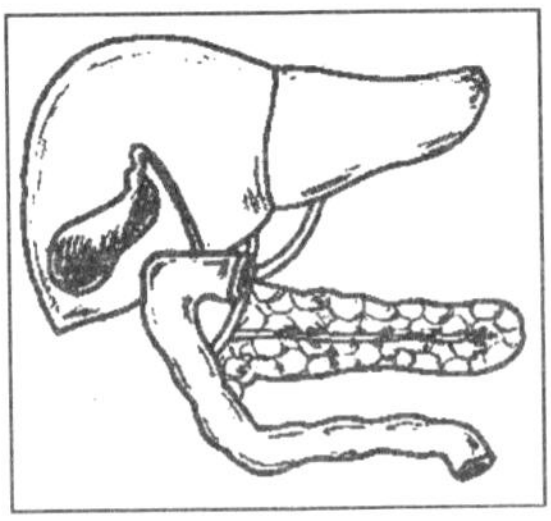

Regulates	:	Blood.
Rules	:	Muscles system, endocrine
Governs	:	Bile and tears
Opens	:	To eyes
Represents	:	Wind Element

Stimulating this point helps in:

(i) Acute and chronic hepatitis.

(ii) Liver stores blood hence it helps in treating:

(a) Anaemia, (b) Dizziness, (c) Cerebrovascular accidents, (d) Painful and irregular periods and (e) Pruritis in skin.

(iii) It opens into eyes.

Treats ophthalmologic diseases

(iv) Helps in digestion.

Intestinal distention, fullness of chest.

(v) Liver meridian energy encircles genitals, hence helps in

(a) Impotence, (b) Infertility and (c) Menstrual problems.

Spleen

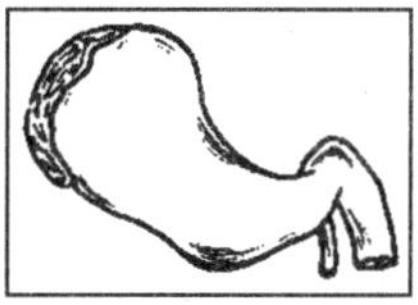

Regulates	:	Transportation and digestion of food.
Rules	:	Soft tissues like fat and covering of the organs
Governs	:	Saliva
Opens	:	To mouth
Represents	:	Earth element

Stimulating this point helps:

(i) Digestion of food.

(ii) Treats obesity (as it transports food and improves metabolism: the deficient working of this organ leads to obesity — one of the main reasons for obesity).

(iii) Strengthens lining of stomach and other digestive organs.

Improves gastrointestinal ulcers.

(iv) Controls gas, flatulence.

(v) Strengthens organs covers.

Prevents hernia development and prolapse.

(vi) Helps in holding blood in vessels

Treats blood diseases

(a) Anaemia b) Prevents haemorrhage.

(vii) Transports energy

(a) Helps in improving immunity

(b) Treats allergies

(c) Skin diseases

Kidney

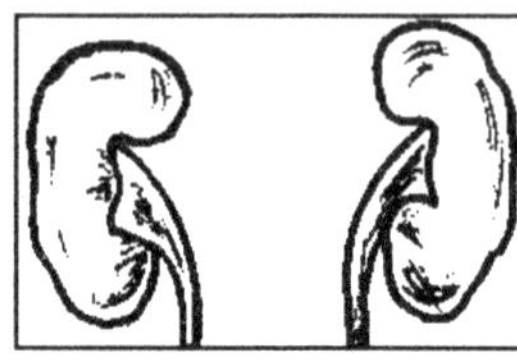

Regulates	:	Bone system (bones, cartilage)
Rules	:	Teeth, bone marrow, head hair
Governs	:	Urine
Opens	:	To ear
Holds	:	Essence of body "Jing" (Helps in passing the hereditary traits maintaining the libido of the individual — Jing is responsible for an individual's constitution and helps in fertility).
Represents	:	Water element

Stimulating this point helps in

(i) Improving function of kidney and treats: (a) Nephritis, (b) Cystitis of kidney, (c) Retention of urine.

(ii) Stores basic essence

(a) Improves reproductive, regeneration system,

(b) Nocturnal pollution.

(iii) Rules bones, teeth and marrow

(a) Helps in arthritis

(b) Improves bone structure, brings in fast healing

(c) Stops recurrence of habitual fractures

(d) Improves loose teeth

(e) Brain is a sea of marrow, improving kidney improves bone marrow which helps in mental and nervous disease.

(f) Helps in treating gout.

(iv) As Kidney energy opens to ear

(a) Helps in reducing deafness, ringing in ear.

(b) Ménière's syndrome (dizziness and vertigo).

(v) As it represents element water

(a) Helps in treating gout.

(b) Helps in reducing excess heat in body.

(c) Hypertension — Burning urine — Bleeding gums.

(d) Epilepsy

(vi) In general increases life energy

Small Intestine

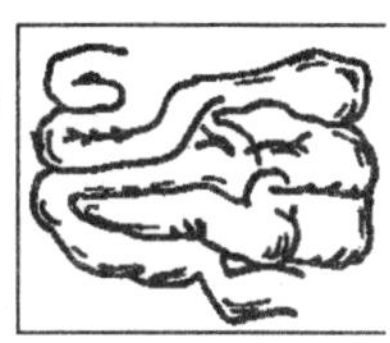

Regulates : Digestion and separating essence from food

Connection : It is connected to heart through meridian

Stimulating this point helps:

(i) Digestive problems: (a) Indigestion, (b) Poor absorption and (c) Abdominal distention.

(ii) Due to connection with heart helps in heart problems like

(a) Palpitation (b) Shortness of breath.

Large Intestine

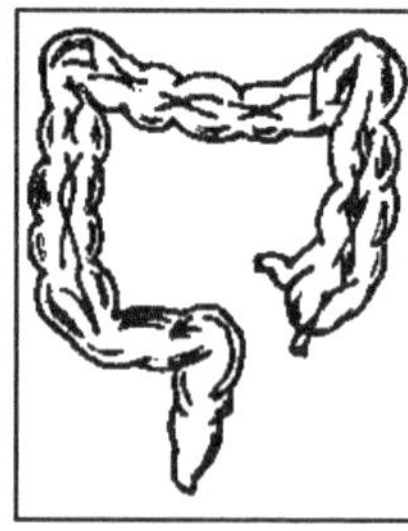

Regulates : Excretion

Connection : It is connected to lungs through meridian.

Stimulating this point helps in:

(i) Excretion problems

(a) Constipation, (b) Remove indigestion and (c) Cures appendicitis.

(ii) Helps in curing irritable bowel syndrome.

(iii) Due to connection with lungs helps in respiratory system.

Stomach

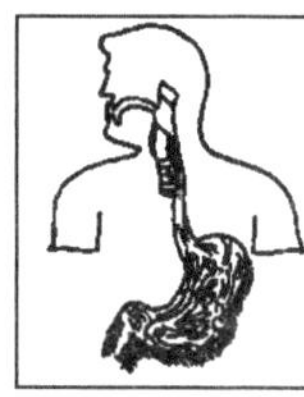

Regulates : Transportation and digestion of food

Connection : To spleen through meridian

Stimulating this point helps in:

(i) Digestion and stomach related problems: (a) Gastric ulcer, (b) Indigestion, (c) Lack of appetite and (d) Gastric-neurosis.

(ii) Calms the stomach

(a) Stops the stomach energy moving upward. This prevents nausea, vomiting.

(b) Stomach meridian travels from the face and ends in frontal part of brain, hence stimulating this point helps in calming the brain and clears thinking.

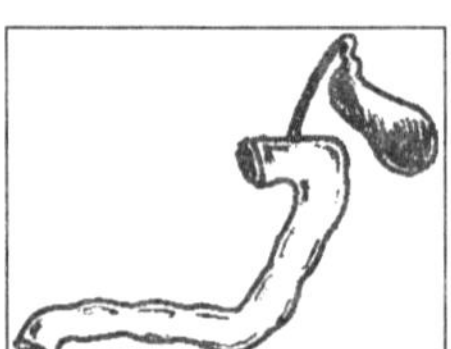

Gall Bladder

Regulates : Storage of bile and mental activity.

Connection : It is connected to liver through meridian.

Stimulating this point helps in:

(i) Proper storage of bile.
Helps digestion.

(ii) Being connected to liver helps in liver-related problems.
(a) Reaches energy to muscle and tendon.
(b) Clears eyesight.

(iii) Gall bladder meridian runs along the temporal region of head around the ears. Hence activating this point helps in:
(a) Relieving headache, (b) Clears head and brings clarity. (c) Helps in deafness and other ear problems.

(iv) Can be used to remove
(a) Gall bladder stone, (b) Cystitis in gall bladder.

Urinary Bladder

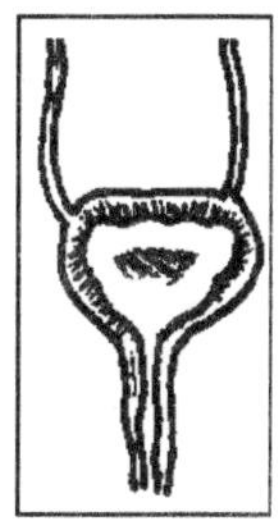

Regulates : Holding urine and flow of urine.

Connection : It is connected to kidney through meridian.

Stimulating this point helps in:

(i) Solving urine-related problems:
(a) Incontinence of urine, (b) Retention of urine and (c) Dribbling urine.

(ii) Bladder stones.

(iii) The urinary bladder meridian has a long course along the dorsal side of the body starting from eyes it goes over the head, neck, the entire back, over the back of thigh and ends at the foot.

Activating this point helps in clearing the meridian energy which helps in treating lumbago, leg pain, headache, insomnia, etc.

5

Five-Element Concept

Five-Elements

OUR body is made of five elements, the *pancha-mahabhutas* as per ancient Indian concept too.

The five elements as per Chinese concept are:

1. Air, 2. Fire, 3. Earth, 4. Metal and 5. Water.

These five elements crystallise in the body as five vital organs, namely:

1. Liver, 2. Heart, 3. Spleen, 4. Lung and 5. Kidney.

They are the main producing yin organs. Each of them is connected to a respective distributing organ, which distributes their energy in the body. The corresponding organs are:

1. Liver : Gall bladder
2. Heart : Small intestine
3. Spleen : Stomach
4. Lung : Large intestine
5. Kidney : Urinary bladder

The energy in these organs moves in a cyclic manner.

These organs are function-specific, each set can be equated to a department.

The functional aspects are discussed in Chinese functional organ notes discussed in the previous chapter.

1. The air/wood element represented by liver, and it is equated to wind, it has the character of:

- Movement, mobility, action. A good liver shows action in the body as well as outside. That is, the person's other organs move and do their functions and the person is active doing his activities when liver functions properly.
- It controls muscles and tendons in the body. Takes care of the sense organ eye. Manages the endocrine in the body.
- Impairment in this causes decrease in movement inside the body and outside the body, i.e. voluntary and involuntary functions.
- Paralysis, infertility, pain in the muscles, lack of growth are all associated with it.

2. The fire element represented by heart and it is equated to heat, it has the character of:

- Warmth, enjoyment, desire, ambition, it represents a warm body, good circulation, and a good spirited mind and emotion.
- It controls circulatory system, mental activity and is in charge of nervous system. The sense organ tongue is conncected to it.
- Impairment in this can cause circulatory problems. An excess can result in bleeding problems, like excess menstrual bleeding, nose bleeding, bleeding piles, hypertension, etc.
- A decrease in heat can cause sluggish circulation, hypotension, etc.
- Further, boils in the body, burning urine, excessive thirst are due to heat.
- Heat also causes mental problems. Less of it will result in depression and more of it in excessive desire, ambition, etc.

- Speech problems are also associated with it as it controls the sense organ tongue.

3. The earth element is represented by spleen, it is equated to dampness, it has the character of:

- Stability, stagnation, settlement, etc. It represents satisfaction, consiousness, thinking, etc.
- It is connected to fertility and giving birth.
- It controls all soft cells in the body like fat, lining of the organs, etc. And is connected to sense of taste.
- An impairment in this can result in obesity, hernia and placid taste in the mouth. This can also cause heaviness, non-healing sores, distension of stomach, etc.

4. The metal element is represented by lung and it is equated to dryness, it has the character of:

- Clarity and a tendency to descend. It is connected with will, determination and perseverance.
- It controls skin fluid mechanism and moistens the skin. It permeates lung and large intestine which are in charge of excretion in the body. It is connected to sense organ nose.
- Impairment in this affects the dispersing and descending functions of lungs and thus causes skin dryness, constipation, reduced urination, dry cough, etc.

5. The water element is represented by kidney and it is equated to coldness, it has the character:

- To flow downwards, cool the system and keeps it tender. It denotes strength, courage and ability to go ahead.
- To some extent it also gives to contraction and stagnation.
- It controls all the skeletal (framework organs of the body) like bones, cartilage, teeth, head hair, nails, etc.

- The sense organ of hearing — the ear, is governed by it.
- Impairment in this causes bone problems resulting in arthritis and spondylosis, hearing loss, a lack of libido, fearfulness, excess urination, etc.

Interaction of Five Elements

The five elements are the basic building blocks in the universe. As human beings are the microcosms in the universe, they are made of the same elements as that present in the universe.

The elements are closely connected with one another. They continuously interact with one another to promote growth as well as to keep each other in check or control.

Creative Cycle

They operate primarily in a promoting, in a creative manner with one element helping the other element in its growth and development.

This is an order of creation, the order is as follows:

1. Wood : promotes fire,
2. Fire : promotes earth,
3. Earth : promotes metal,
4. Metal : promotes water,
5. Water : promotes wood,

Thus in nature we find from wood comes fire, by burning of fire earth is made, earth stores the metal in it, the internal cool metal stores up the water.

In the same way liver promotes the working of heart, the heart fire helps in the digestion in stomach and spleen, the spleen's assimilation helps the working of lung and large intestine, the lung energy acts on the kidney and helps in maintaining the water balance.

Thus the promoting element is the mother and promoted element is the son.

Example : Liver is the mother of heart and heart is the mother of spleen. Heart is the son of liver and spleen the son of heart.

Controlling Cycle

Apart from the promoting cycle, elements are subjected to a controlling cycle. In this, one element acts on another to control its excess action. This controlling action is required to keep the element in check.

The counteracting cycle acts in the following way:

1. Wood : controls earth,
2. Earth : controls water,
3. Water : controls fire
4. Fire : controls metal,
5. metal : controls wood

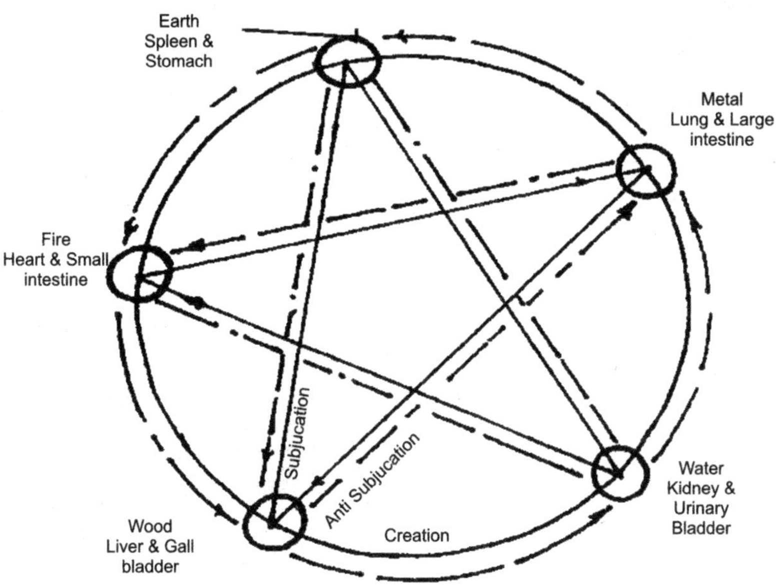

Translating this into human organs.

1. Liver : controls spleen,	4. Heart : controls lungs
2. Spleen : controls kidney,	5. Lung : controls liver.
3. Kidney : controls heart,	

Thus if heart is in excess resulting in hypertension it can be rectified by treating kidney point.

If spleen and stomach are in excess resulting in obesity it can be rectified by treating liver point and improving it.

Anti-Creative Cycle

Generally the action within the five elements is of promoting and controlling, and the organ and function are maintained in harmony and in control aiding general well-being of the body.

However, due to some physiological reasons or pathological reasons the cycle can be reversed.

Thus we can have situation in which

1. Water : promotes metal,	1. Kidney : promotes lung,
2. Metal : promotes earth,	2. Lung : promotes spleen,
3. Earth : promotes fire,	3. Spleen : promotes heart,
4. Fire : promotes wood,	4. Heart : promotes liver,
5. Wood : promotes water,	5. Liver : promotes kidney.

This cycle is not good for the health of the human body and this results in disease, or this state may result because of some disease affecting the body.

It is the case of son promoting mother which is not natural.

Example: A case of fire promoting wood or heart in excess in comparison to liver will cause damage to the liver in bringing in some heat disorder, like swelling, inflammation or jaundice.

Anti-Controlling Cycle

This is also a reverse cycle. Instead of one element controlling and helping to co-ordinate another element, it may go to controlling in reverse order which may lead to destruction.

The cycle may get reversed due to various physiological and pathological reasons.

Thus we can have a state of:

1. Wood : controlling metal,	1. Liver : controlling lung,
2. Water : controlling earth,	2. Lung : controlling spleen,
3. Metal : controlling fire,	3. Kidney : controlling heart,
4. Earth : controlling wood,	4. Spleen : controlling liver,
5. Fire : controlling water,	5. Heart : controlling kidney.

Example: A common problem is fire acting on water. Increased fire can result in heat problems in the body while decreased water may result in skeleton problems like lumbago, spondylosis, etc.

The five-element information is discussed here in brief so that while treating the ear points and the respective organs, in cases which do not respond to ear reflexology alone, these cycles will help to decide the modalities of treatment.

6

Therapeutics

EAR reflex points provide an admirable tool for treatment of various health disorders. Further, as the entire body is represented in a small unit as ear, this can be taken to advantage and only a small area has to be examined and treated. Apart from the reflex points the potent master therapeutic points help to bring quick results in the body chemistry and make the treatment effective. However, clear understanding of diagnosis and accuracy in effecting the treatment are necessary to get good results.

Examination of the Ear

Before starting the ear therapy the ear has to be thoroughly examined. The examination is to find the problem areas and then correlate it with the corresponding parts of the body.

For examination the ear should be seen in a good light. Natural light is preferable, alternatively a good torchlight can be used.

The ear has to be palpated and slightly massaged with hand before starting the examination. This is to allow the blood to flow and bring out the pain referrals.

In a particularly non-reactive ear, the zero point can be pricked or given firm pressure to bring out other pain referrals to the fore.

A probe can be used for inspection. It can be an electrical probe or an ordinary steel or wooden probe, or even a matchstick also can serve as a probe.

For some particular examination like blood circulation or checking the neuroglia at a particular spot or numbness in some parts of the body, a hot or cold probe can be used.

The folds of the ear have to be lifted and upturned to examine clearly the inner parts.

Note the ear to be examined is the one on the same side of the problem, that is the homo/ipsilateral side. Thus for gall bladder we have to check the right side while for pancreas the left side of the ear has to be checked.

The ear has to be examined for:

1. Colour change
2. Texture
3. Deposits
4. Pain and Tenderness
5. Inflammation
6. Numbness

1. Colour change : Dark spots indicate stagnation. Red spots indicate heat and inflammation. White spots with fur indicate diseased state of organ. Black decolouration shows metabolism is not proper.

2. Texture : Shining elastic ear represents good health. Hard ear represents calcification of the blood vessels. Pale and thin ear represents weak health and a weak kidney.

3. Deposits : White furs indicate disease and degeneration. Red congested papules indicate congestion of blood. Black protruding papules or thick lines indicate stagnation

		of energy. Oily deposits indicate good internal secretion. A dry ear indicates internal secretions are getting dried.
4. Pain and tenderness	:	Pain and tenderness at a particular point indicates disturbance of the corresponding part or organ of the body.
5. Inflammation	:	Pain along with inflammation indicates heat conditions in the corresponding part.
6. Numbness	:	Due to constriction of arteries and other reasons the corresponding part of the body will be having a dysfunction.

ORDER OF EXAMINATION

1. Mildly press with the probe uniformly the entire ear. One can start with shenmen/zero point. A firm pressure if evicts pain can be kept as base referral point.

   Start the examination with conchae-cavum and cymba conchae. This will help to gauge the status of the organs.
2. Then move to anti-helix and examine the vertebrae and brain from anti-tragus to lower portion of inferior crus of anti-helix.
3. Examine then scapha and the lobe.
4. Examine then the helix in detail. Many referral points in helix will match with the corresponding points found inside as helix represents the outermost sheath of the body.

Use of Different Probes

1. **Normal probe :** Used for detecting uniformly all problems.
2. **Hot probe :** Will help to show and treat non-reactive spots which are numb or having very little vascular movements.

3. **Cold probe :** Will help to show and treat over-reactive spots. These instruments also act as good tools to find the reactive points — spots which are inflamed, overactive and very painful.

4. **Electronic probe :** The tender spots react sharply to an electronic probe which is translated to sound. Thus a sharper sound is heard in reactive spots. These instruments act as good tools to find the reactive points and treat the same.

Modalities of Treatment

After diagnosis both by physical examination and taking case history of the patient, the points to be treated are to be decided. At times if the problem is not severe, there may not be any immediate tell-tale signs. Then diagnosis should be made by hearing the case history of the patient and carefully search for the reactive points with a probe.

DIFFERENT METHODS OF TREATMENT

On understanding the reflex information the ear emits of different body parts and also the therapeutic master points present in the auricle, the treatment of these points has to be effected.

The main objective of the treatment is to stimulate these reflective and reactive points. The stimulation of these remote points produces a curing electromagnetic reflex in the corresponding body part and cures the affliction. Thus ear can be used as a remote control very similar to how we use our remote to operate the T.V. If human brain can produce a remote to control a machine it is not at all far-fetching to accept that the nature has given us a remote in the auricle.

The stimulation can be brought about:

1. By manual stimulation,
2. By acupuncture, and

3. By applying small objects like seeds, button magnets, pellets, etc., on the reactive points.

By Manual Stimulation

(a) **Finger massage**: This is the easiest yet effective method of treatment. The auricle is massaged gently, starting from the conchae and progressively moving to the anti-helix, scapha, the triangular fossa and finally the helix. The folds should be lifted and examined for any reactive point. At places of reactive area more stress should be given and pressure applied steadily and firmly. Stimulate the point by rotatory motion from time to time. Note for tenderness. Minimum of four to five times a day till the tenderness in the place is removed.

(b) **Massage with a probe**: On deducing the reactive points, probes made of steel, wood or even toothpick, matchstick can be substituted as probe and the points can be massaged or given pressure alternatively.

Acupuncture

The most effective method of treating the ear is by acupuncture. Fine filiform sterilised needles are inserted on the treatment point and kept in place for a minimum period of twenty minutes and the procedure repeated daily or alternate days for ten days.

Certain guidelines have to be followed in acupuncture procedures:

- The needles used are fine filiform steel needles of 30 to 32 gauge. Gold and silver needles are not used routinely, but when used, gold helps in tonification and silver helps in sedation. The needle length does not exceed generally more than half inch. Generally steel needles are used. The ear has to be gently massaged to help the energy to flow and cleaned with an antiseptic with the help of cotton wool before insertion of needle. The tender points can be searched either with a probe made of wood or steel or with an electronic point finder. Ear is a soft part of the body, upper $4/5^{th}$ made of cartilage and lower $1/5^{th}$ made of soft tissue. While needling care has to be taken and the cartilage is not to be penetrated. The needling can be done vertically or horizontally covering more points at a time or obliquely depending on the place where the needling is to be done in the ear.

- At one time not more than three or four needles are inserted in one ear. At the same point more than one needle can be inserted in different angles to bring correct reactions in treating cases like paralysis or acute pain, etc.
- The needles have to be sterilised by simple procedure of antiseptic solutions like spirit or Dettol, etc.
- It is safer to use individual needles (separate set) for each patient or disposable needles.
- The needles are kept *in situ* for a minimum period of twenty minutes, as per the case the time period can be extended to one hour.
- Ear problems are tackled on ipsilateral/homolateral side. That is the problems on left side are tackled on left ear and one on the right side are tackled on the right ear.
- Generally locomotor problems are tackled on the same ear, while organ problems are tackled on both the ears.
- Needle pecking is also a way of treating by needles, when with the help of small plum blossom needles (a bunch of needles attached to the end of a stick) the ear is activated for the "chi" or energy to flow.
- The needles are at times stimulated with electrical stimulation. This is especially so for treating addictions. Small electrically operated machines ranging from 4 to 9 volts are used. The needles are plugged on to the machine with the help of wires having clips for

attachment. The stimulation is given for a period ranging from 10 to 30 minutes.

- The stimulation also can be given from body to ear. In that case the positive electrode is plugged to the ear and the negatives to the body for stimulation.
- Negative electrode is plugged to the ear and positive to the body for sedative purpose. Normal frequency can be 80 to 100 hertz. But for anaesthesia high frequency of 2000 hertz is given. For certain problems low frequency ranging between 5 and 20 hertz is used. The intensity for stimulation is set between 20 and 80 microamps depending on the tolerence of the patient treated.
- Press needles are also used. They are small mini needles attached with a stopper so that the needle does not slip into the skin completely. They also come with an adhesive tape which can be stuck along with the needle. Such press needles are left in the ear for a period of one week. Care has to be taken that the patient is not prone to infection problems. As the ear has comparatively less blood vessels healing sometimes becomes a problem. If the infection happens antibiotics have to be given.

Fixing seeds, Steel Pellets, Small Button Magnets

They can be fixed to the reactive or problem effective point with an adhesive tape or plaster and pressed from time to time which can also show good curing effect.

The seeds with their natural energy also help in treating the point, even without resorting to constant pressing.

Colour therapy can be also used to select the colour of seeds.

Red seeds are for tonification.

Black seeds for sedation.

Generally small seeds like mustard, fenugreek seeds (*methi*), etc. are used.

Evaluating the Treatment Points

This can be decided using:

1. The reflex points.
2. Therapeutic points.
3. Points as per Chinese Meridian Therapy.
4. Points of five elements (their subjugation and anti-subjugation principles).
5. Points as per Western medicine.

1. Initially the reflex points have to be found which can be distinguished by pain, tenderness, decolouration, swelling, growth of furs, nodules, red or black dots, etc.
2. The theraputic points can be added depending upon the problem.

   If sedation is required - Ear shenmen point can be used.

   If action is required - Ear adrenal point can be used.

   If pain relief is required - Ear thalamus point can be used.

   If asthma problem - Ear Dingchaun point can be used.
3. Further Chinese meridian (energy flowing) information is taken into account. For this both functional aspect (as given in separate notes on each organ functional aspect) and area traversed by meridian are taken into account to decide points to be selected for treatment.
4. Also the five-element theory where each organ is represented by an element and the rules of the controlling cycle rules are taken into account to treat a problem, especially the one which does not respond well to reflex point and therapeutic point treatment, more so the chronic ones where the problem has seeped and rooted into the body.

For example:

Liver represents wood	: Wind
Heart represents heat	: Fire
Spleen represents earth	: Dampness
Lung represents metal	: Dryness
Kidney represents water	: Coldness

A person having more heat can be treated with water, i.e. kidney. A person having more water can be treated with fire, i.e. heart. As water subjugates fire and heat subjugates water.

5. Treatment is also decided as per Western medicine concepts. Thus urine problems are treated through kidney points. Circulatory problems through heart point.

Precautions

Don't do press needling of pregnant woman.

Don't do ear needling on patients who are using cardiac pacemaker.

Make sure the person is not prone to infection before administering press needles.

Press needles can be inserted after few rounds of treatment when person's immunity is spruced up.

Don't treat an excessively tired, hungry, famished patient or patient after heavy meals.

If the patient feels dizzy or nervous ask him to lie down and rest when the needles are inserted.

In case of infection treat the patient with antibiotic.

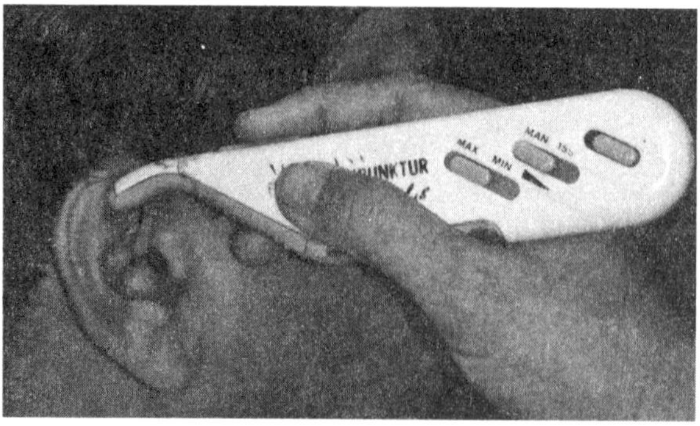

Treatment by electronic probe

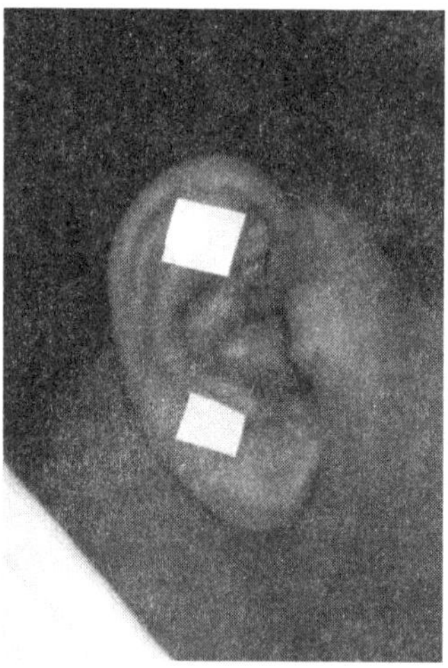

Treatment by fixing seeds by pellets

Treatment by Acupuncture

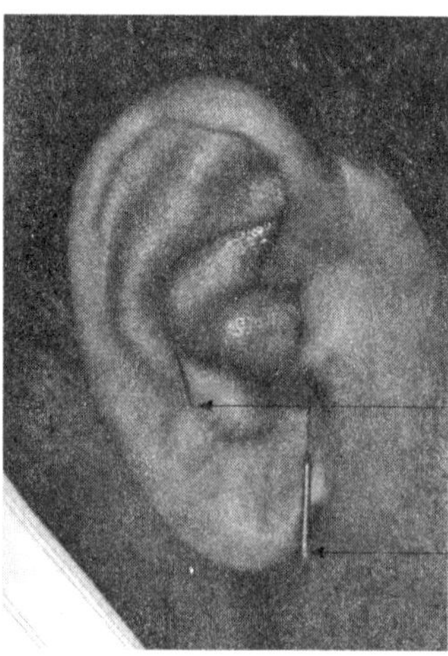

Liver Point

Endocrine Point

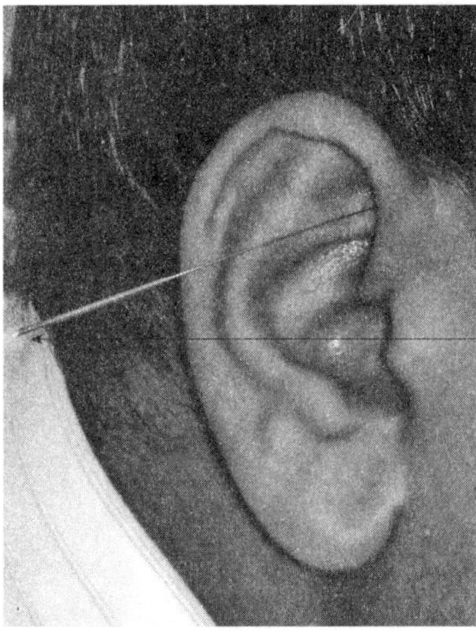

Sympathetic Nerve Point

Physiognomy of the Ear

Understanding the physique and physiology of a person by observing the ear was an age-old science. The ear almost acts like finger print in identifying and understanding the person. No two persons' ears are alike, even the right and left ears are slightly different. The ear continuously grows as the person ages.

As per Chinese acupuncture science the *"chi"* or the energy of the kidney opens in the ear. It is found the ear resembles or depicts the kidney. From the ear we can gauge the size and shape of the kidney.

Now kidneys are repositories of genetic wealth handed over from our parents. Thus a good-sized ear shows strong kidneys and good genetic strength inherited.

An ideal ear should be round at the top, wide in the middle, tapered and long towards the lobe like Lord Buddha's ear.

From the ear we can find the circulatory, nervous, digestive strength of our system.

Circulatory

The outer rim, helix, represents the circulation in the body. If the rim is well built and thick it reveals good circulation. The person will have regulated body temperature. His extremities will be warm and well nourished.

A good circulation also gets translated in the nature. He will have the ability to circulate or move with a wide variety of people amiably. He will have a stable centred personality and easily make friends.

People with narrow rim or no rim tend to be suspicious of others and keep to themselves.

Nervous System

The nervous system is represented by the internal rim or anti-helix. A strong anti-helix and anti-tragus shows well-developed nervous system. The person can be intelligent and analytical. He will be a thinker getting insight into things.

Digestive System

Conchae and the crus of helix shows the strength of the digestive system. A deep wide conchae with well-pronounced crus shows a good ability to digest. This ability gets translated in the mental level. Such a person is able to digest life. He can face life as well as enjoy it.

Earlobe

A person with ample earlobe has good fortune and understanding of life. They are flexible to life's circumstances. They get involved in profession which has dealings with people. People with attached earlobes have a narrow view of life and tend to move towards technical profession. However people with small earlobes can also be focused having drive and ambition but their understanding of people will not be broad hence may face emotional surprises.

7

Treatments

Treatment for Disorders

1. Respiratory disorders
2. Circulatory disorders
3. Digestive disorders
4. Gynaecological disorders
5. Psychological disorders
6. Kidney and urinary disorders
7. Liver disorders
8. Back pain and arthritis
9. Neurological disorders
10. Eyesight disorders
11. Hearing disorders
12. Glandular and sexual disorders
13. Skin and allergies
14. Migraine and headache
15. Drug addiction — (Alcohol addiction, smoking addiction), food addiction (obesity)
16. Common problems with Single point remedy — knee pain, dental pain, sciatica, constipation, blood pressure, insomnia, diabetes, impotence, appendicitis, asthma attack, stomach upset, urticaria, tonsillitis, vertigo, hernia, concentration improvement, sneezing bouts.

Respiratory

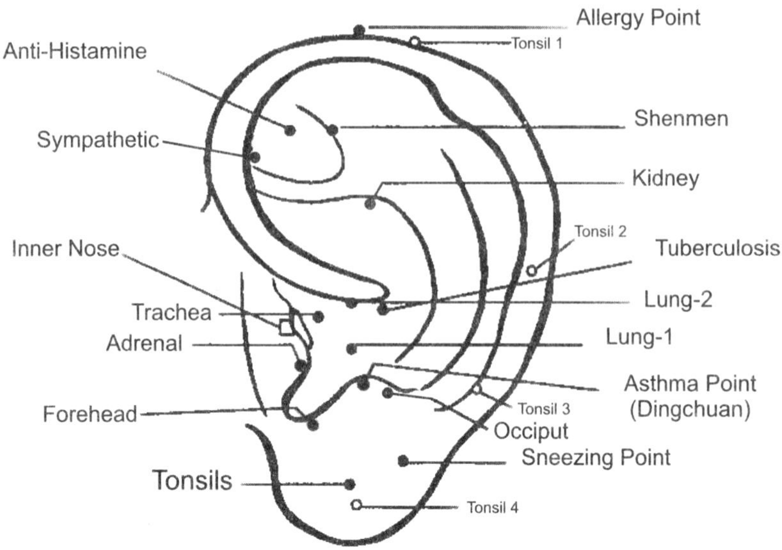

Disease	*Primary Points*	*Secondary Points*
Cough	Lung 1&2, Pharynx, Adrenal Point	Sympathetic
Common Cold	Internal nose, Lung 1 & 2	Forehead, adrenal
Sinus	Occiput, Forehead, Lung	Adrenal, sympathetic
Asthma	Dingchuan, Antihista-mine, Shenmen, Adrenal	Lung, Kidney
Broncho pneumonia	Trachea, Endocrine, Lung	Dingchuan, Thalamus
Tuberculosis	Lung, Adrenal gland, Tuberculosis point	Kidney, Spleen, Zero point
Sneezing	Sneezing point, Lung, Brain stem	Internal nose
Tonsillitis	Helix 1-6, Tonsillitis (L 8), Ear apex to bleed, occiput.	Sympathetic

Circulatory

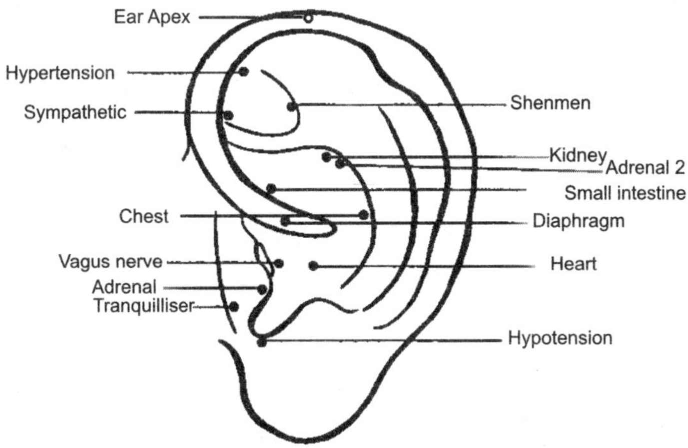

Disease	*Primary Points*	*Secondary Points*
Hypertension	Groove in the back of ear, Heart, Shenmen, Ear apex to bleed	Tranquilliser, Kidney
Hypotension	Hypotension point, Adrenal Heart	Sympathetic, Spleen, Liver.
Angina	Heart, Sympathetic, Chest, Stomach,Vagus nerve, Shenmen	Small intestine, Kidney
Palpitation	Zero point, sympathetic, Heart	Thalamus point
Anaemia	Heart, Endocrine, Spleen, Diaphragm	Liver
Cardiac arrest	Heart, Chest, Adrenal 1 & 2, Endocrine glands, Shenmen	Thalamus, Spleen
Cold hands & feet numbness	Heart, Adrenal, Endocrine	Pituitary, Spleen
Arteriosclerosis	Heart, Kidney, Small intestine, Adrenal	Endocrine, Sympathetic

Digestive

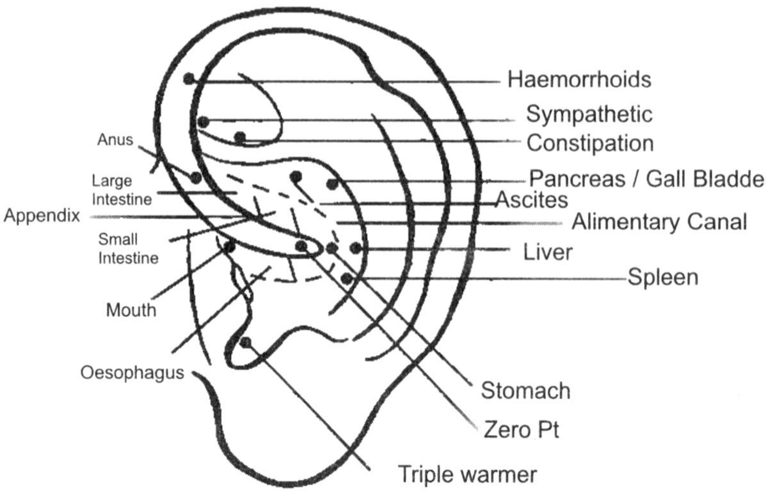

Disease	*Primary Points*	*Secondary Points*
Nausea	St., Shenmen, Zero point	Oesophagus
Diarrhoea	Large intestine, Small intestine, Rectum	Abdomen, Spleen
Constipation	Constipation, L.I., Triple warmer, rectum	Sympathetic, Stomach
Indigestion	Stomach, Pancreas, Spleen, Liver	L.I., Sympathetic
Abdominal	Ascites, St., Zero point	Sympathetic
Distension	Triple warmer, Rectum	Abdomen
Gastric Ulcer	St., Sympathetic, Shenmen	Lung, Spleen, Duodenum
Acidity	St., Zero point, Tranquilliser	Spleen, Shenmen
Gas problem	St., Gall bladder, Spleen	Darwins tubercle, Zero pt., Vagus nerve

Haemorrhoids	Haemorrhoids, Rectum	Sympathetic
Appendix	Appendix, Shenmen, Zero point, L.I.	Clavicle, Darwins tubercle, Shenmen
Irritable bowel Syndrome	St., Small intestine, Large intestine, Rectum	Abdomen, Sympathetic
Diabetes	Pancreas, Spleen, Endocrine, Adrenal,	Liver, Sympathetic
Hernia	Spleen, Abdomen, Corresponding body area	Sympathetic

Gynaecological

Disease	*Primary Points*	*Secondary Points*
Infertility	Uterus, Ovary, Kidney, Endocrine, Adrenal	Brain stem, Sympathetic
Irregular menstruation	Ovary, Spleen, Kidney, Thalamus point, Adrenal	Liver, Sympathetic
White discharge	Vagina, Zero point, Shenmen	Brain stem, Kidney
Labour Induction	Uterus, Abdomen, Pelvic girdle, Thalamus, Lumbar spine	Spleen, Zero point
Lactation	Mammary gland, Endocrine	Spleen, Sympathetic
Menopause	Ovary, Uterus, Kidney	Endocrine
Ovarian/ Uterus tumor	Ovary, Uterus, Endocrine, Shenmen, Thalamus point	Heart, Zero point
Premenstrual problem	Ovary (Brain Pt.), Ovary (at Helix crus), Shenmen, Uterus, Kidney	Sympathetic

Gynaecological

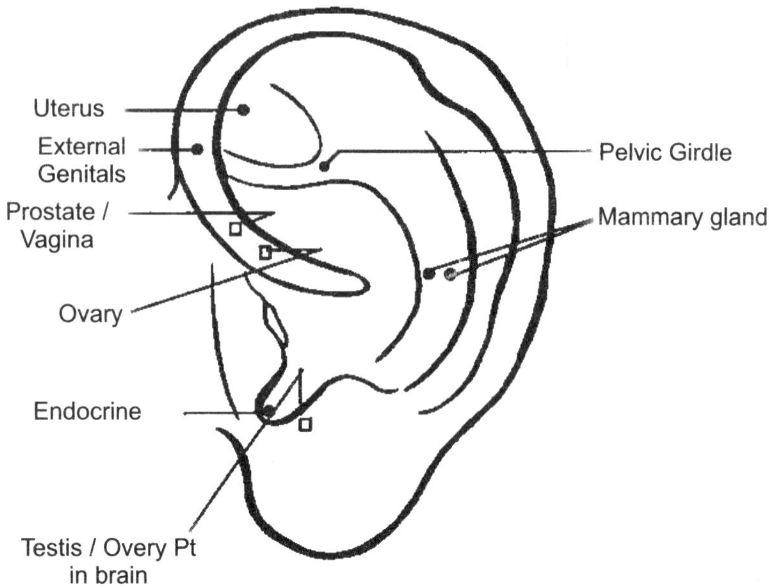

Psychological

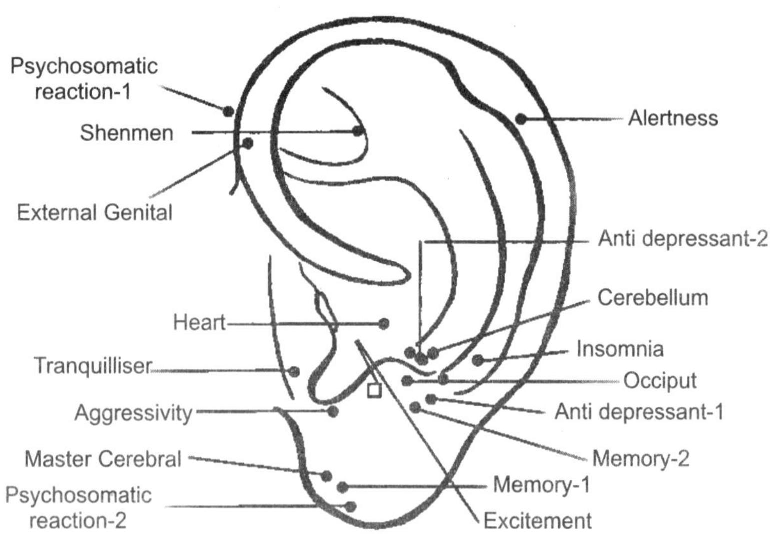

Psychological

Disease	*Primary Points*	*Secondary Points*
Anxiety	Master cerebral, Tranquilliser, Zero point, Shenmen	Heart, Vagus nerve
Depression	Anti-depressant 1 & 2, Root of helix, Master cerebral	Brain stem, Heart
Hysteria	Subcortex, Thalamus, Occiput Zero point, Shenmen	Small occipital nerve
Schizo-phrenia	Master cerebral, Shenmen, Heart, Thalamus	Kidney, Occiput
Memory problem	Memory 1, Memory 2, Heart, Master cerebral	Shenmen
Irritability	Aggressivity, Zero point, Shenmen, Liver (ear apex)	Thalamus point
Insomnia	Insomnia 1 &2, Tranquilliser, Zero point, Shenmen, Occiput	Brain Stem
Chronic fatigue	Adrenal point, Anti-depressant, Alertness	Stomach & spleen
Drowsiness	Excitement, Alertness, Tranquilliser	Spleen, liver
Jet lag	Insomnia, Shenmen, Zero point	Pineal gland
Excess activity	Sympathetic, Thalamus, External genital, Kidney	Shenmen
Stress & strain	Psychosomatic Reaction 1 & 2, Tranquilliser, Zero point	Shenmen, Adrenal

Kidney & Urinary Disorders

Disease	*Primary Points*	*Secondary Points*
Nephritis	Kidney, Occiput, Clavicle, Shenmen, sympathetic	Spleen
Kidney stones	Kidney, Ureter, Urinary bladder, Shenmen, Heart	Thalamus, Zero point
Urinary infection	Ureter, Bladder, Urethra, Shenmen, Zero point	Adrenal, Spleen, Occiput
Bladder control	Kidney, Bladder, Zero point, Spleen	Sympathetic
Bed-wetting	Vagus nerve, Bladder, Kidney	Shenmen
Frequent urination	Kidney, Bladder, Adrenal, Spleen	Sympathetic

Kidney and Urinary Disorders

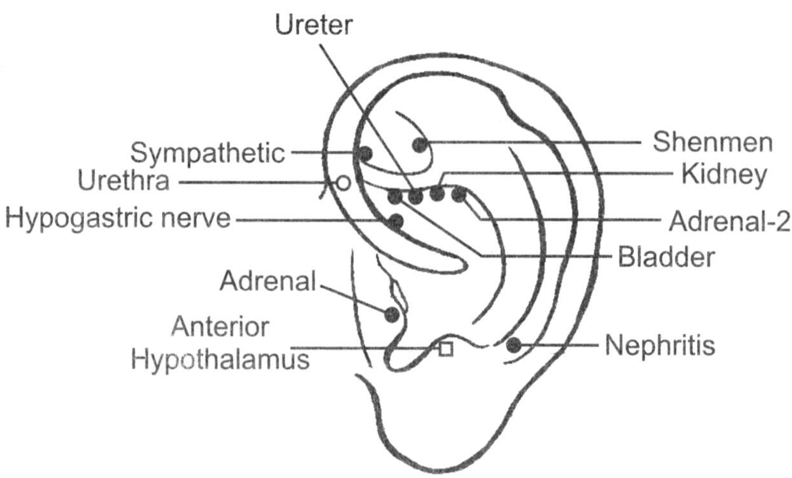

Liver Disorders

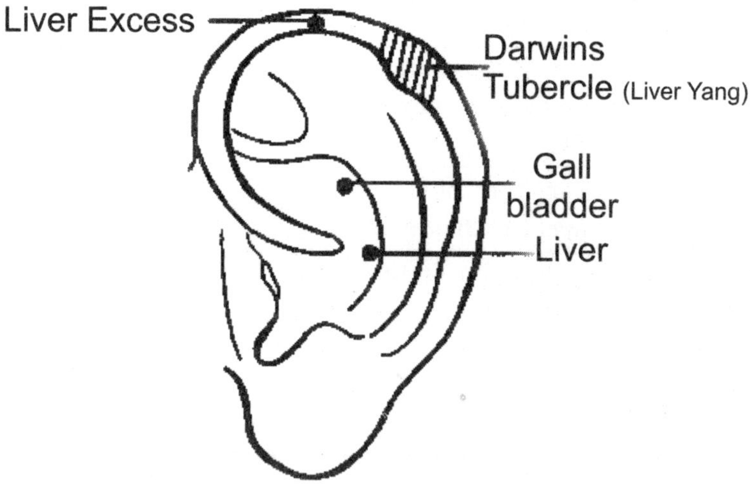

Back pain and arthritis

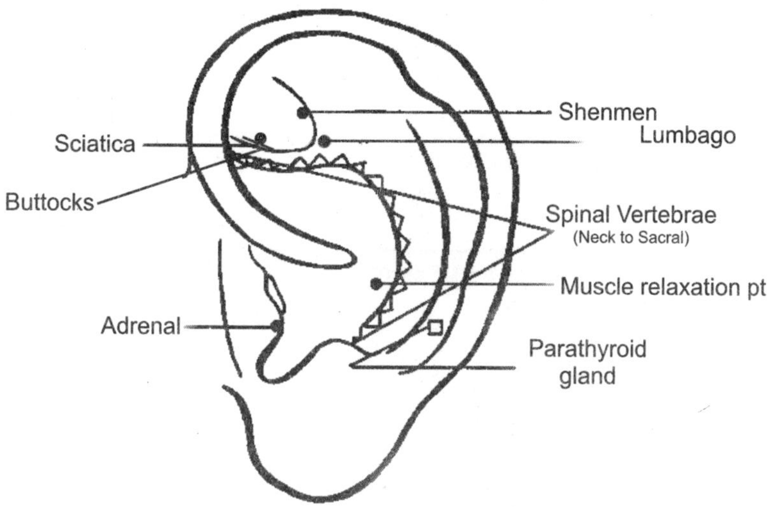

Liver Disorders

Disease	*Primary Points*	*Secondary Points*
Cirrhosis	Liver, Darwins tubercle, Shenmen, Sympathetic, Endocrine	Lung
Hepatitis	Liver, Zero point, Shenmen, Spleen, Darwins tubercle	Gall bladder, St.
Gall Stones	Gall bladder, Zero point, Liver, Endocrine	Lung, Sympathetic

Back pain and Arthritis

Disease	*Primary Points*	*Secondary Points*
Back pain	Corresponding spine-related part in anti-helix, Thalamus point, Muscle relaxation point	Kidney, Adrenal point
Osteoarthritis	Corresponding body area, Kidney, Adrenal, Shenmen, Endocrine	Thalamus point
Rheumatoid arthritis	Corresponding body parts Helix 1-6, Shenmen, Allergy point	Adrenal point
Sciatica	Sciatic nerve, Buttocks, Lumbago, Occiput	Thalamus point
Tennis elbow	Elbow, Forearm, Zero pt.	Shenmen
Muscle cramp/ Sports injuries	Corresponding body area, Muscle relaxation point, Parathyroid gland	Spleen, Cerebellum

Neurological Pain

Disease	*Primary Points*	*Secondary Points*
Epilepsy	Shenmen, Zero point, Thalamus, Occiput, Subcortex (upper half)	Small occipital nerve, Spleen
Cerebral Palsy	Brain stem, Master cerebral, Zero point	Shenmen
Bell's Palsy	Face, Facial nerve, Zero pt., Adrenal	Shenmen
Hyperactivity (Pituitary pt.),	Thyroid control Thyroid gland, Master cerebral	Brain stem, Occiput, Kidney
Stroke	Corresponding body area, Adrenal, pituitary, Master cerebral	Endocrine pt.
Post-Polio Syndrome	Corresponding body parts, Adrenal, Brain stem, Master cerebral Endocrine	Thalamus
Tremors	Spinal motor neurons, Cerebellum, ACTH hormone, Adrenal	Shenmen
Multiple sclerosis	Corresponding body area, Brain stem, Zero point, Thymus gland, Vitality point	

Neurological

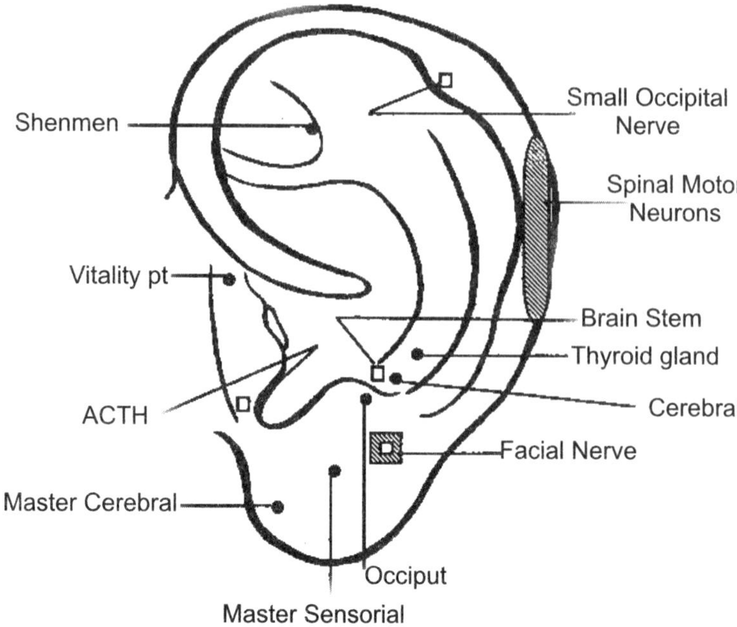

Eyesight

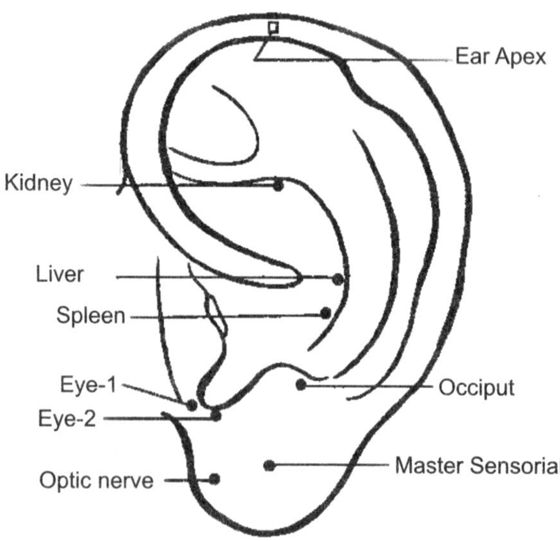

Eyesight Disorders

Disease	*Primary Points*	*Secondary Points*
Conjunctivitis Ear apex to be bled	Eye-1, Eye-2, Eye, Liver,	Kidney
Glaucoma	Eye-1 & 2, Shenmen, Eye, Liver, Spleen	
Stye	Eye, Liver, Spleen	Shenmen
Eye irritation	Eye-1 & 2, Endocrine pt., Ear apex, Sensorial point.	Shenmen
Myopia	Eye-1 & 2, Optic nerve, Kidney	Occiput

Hearing Disorders

Disease	*Primary Points*	*Secondary Points*
Vertigo	Inner ear, Cerebellum, Kidney	Thalamus point
Ear infection	Inner ear, External ear, Spleen, Shenmen	Zero point
Motion sickness	Inner ear, St., Zero point	Shenmen
Sensorial deafness	Inner ear, Auditory nerve, Temporal Cortex, Line of sound, Kidney, Occiput	G.B. & Triple warmer
Sudden deafness	Inner ear, Brain stem, Zero point	Shenmen
Tinnitus (ringing in ear)	Inner ear, Auditory nerve, Master sensorial, Adrenal	Triple warmer, Kidney

Hearing Disorder

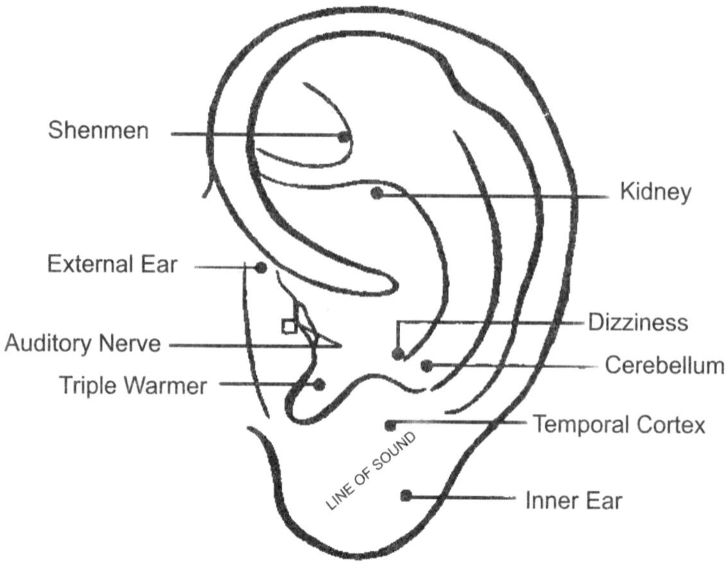

Glandular and Sexual Disorders

Diesase	*Primary Points*	*Secondary Points*
Goitre	Thyroid control, Thyroid gland, Endocrine point, Adrenal	Shenmen
Dwarfism	Subcortex (upper half), Endocrine point, Ovaries or testes	Kidney
Prostatitis	Prostate, Testis, Pelvic girdle, Bladder, Kidney	Zero point
Testitis	Testis, External genitals, Shenmen, Endocrine	Spleen
Impotency, Frigidity	Sexual desire, External genitals, Ovaries or testes, Uterus, Kidney	Sympathetic, Master cerebral

Rash in external genitals	External genitals, Skin disorder, Master sensorial, Endocrine, Lung	
Sexual compulsiveness	Sexual compulsion, Aggressivity point, Tranquilliser, Master cerebral	Heart
Leucorrhoea	Uterus, Internal secretion, Ovary	

Glandular & Sexual Disorders

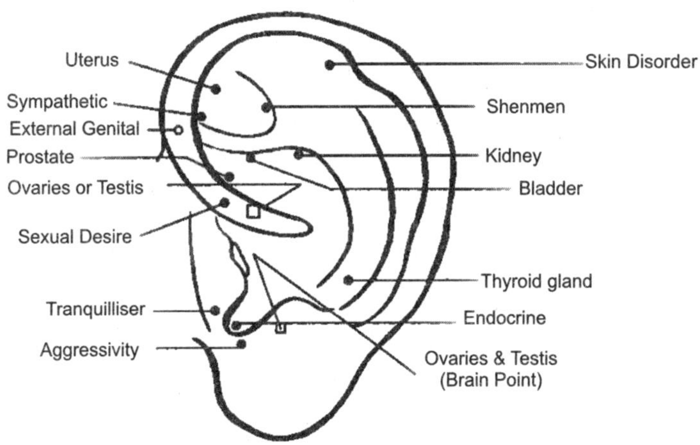

Skin & Allergies

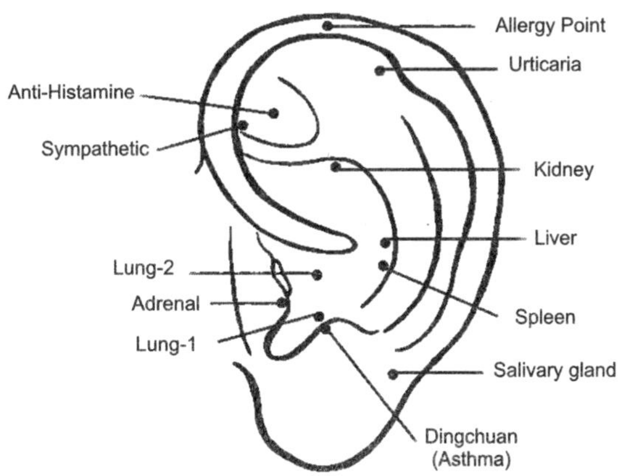

Skin and Allergies

Disease	*Primary Points*	*Secondary Points*
Allergies	Apex of ear (prick to bleed), Thymus gland, Thyroid gland, Asthma, Antihistamine	Sympathetic, Shenmen
Urtricaria	Corresponding body area, Urticaria point	Shenmen, Zero point
Psoriasis	Lung, Spleen, Master cerebral, Master sensorial	
Acne	Face, Urticaria, Lung, Zero point, External genitals	Shenmen
Boils	Corresponding body area, Lung 1 & 2, Zero point, Spleen	Endocrine
Hair loss (Alopecia)	Lung 1 & 2, Kidney, Occiput, Forehead, Lung, Internal secretion, Occiput	Shenmen, Zero point, Kidney, Bladder
Leucoderma	Adrenal gland, points of the corresponding area	

Migraine and Headache

Disease	*Primary Points*	*Secondary Points*
Migraine	Forehead, Shenmen, Sympathetic, Thalamus point, Small occipital nerve, Tranquilliser	Liver, Kidney
Headache	Occiput, Subcortex, Shenmen, Heart, Psychosomatic, Reaction 1 & 2, Master cerebral	Kidney, Sympathetic

Migraine and Headache

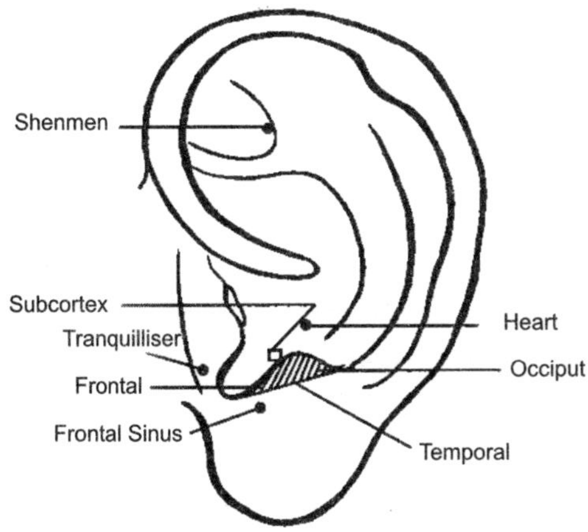

Addiction

Addictions like alcohol, drug, smoking, food are treated effectively by ear reflex points either by Acupuncture or Acupressure.

Addiction	Points along addiction axis line — 1st axis line points: Shenmen, Kidney, Zero point, lung, Brain 2nd axis line points: Sympathetic, Master cerebral
Specific addiction	
Alcohol addiction	Ascites point, Liver, Brain, Thirst point
Drug addiction	Mouth, Heart, Stomach, Aggressivity point, Master cerebral
Smoking addiction	Nicotine point, Lung 1 & 2, Anti-depressant point, Master cerebral
Food addiction	Mouth, Appetite control, Zero point Anti-depressant, Brain, Adrenal gland
Obesity	Good results are obtained in controlling obesity and regulating by auricular stimulation
If due to over-eating	Appetite control, Mouth (hunger point), Heart, Shenmen, Master cerebral

If due to metabolism disorder	Stomach, Spleen, Liver, Abdomen
If due to hormone disorder	Endocrine, Subcortex, Zero point, Occiput, Anti-depressant

The points which are tender can also be treated electrically using low frequency electricity from 10 to 80 hertz.

Addiction Drug, Alcohol, Smoking, food

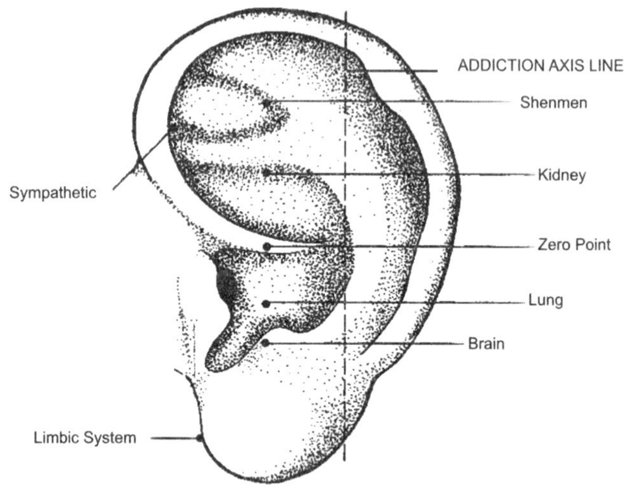

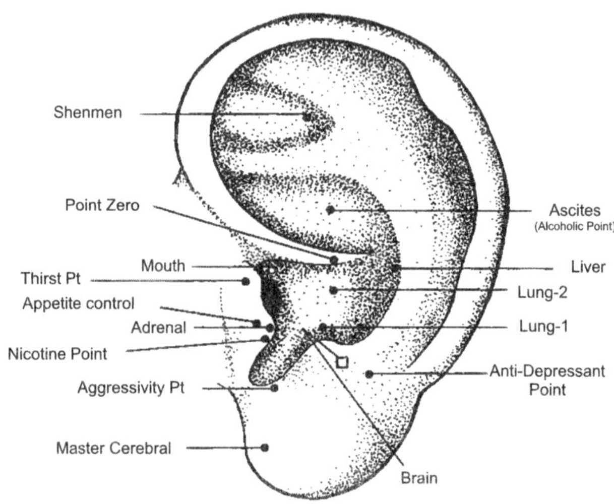

Common Problems — Single Point Remedy

Knee Pain

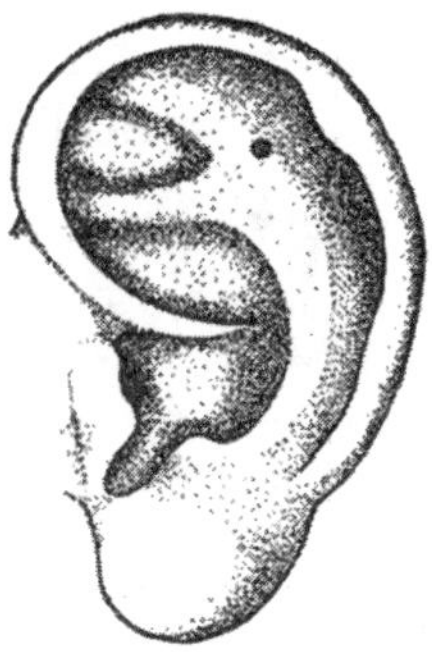

Dental Pain

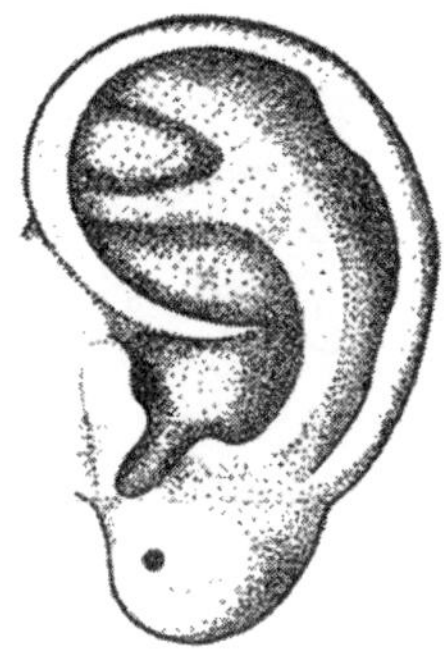

Sciatica

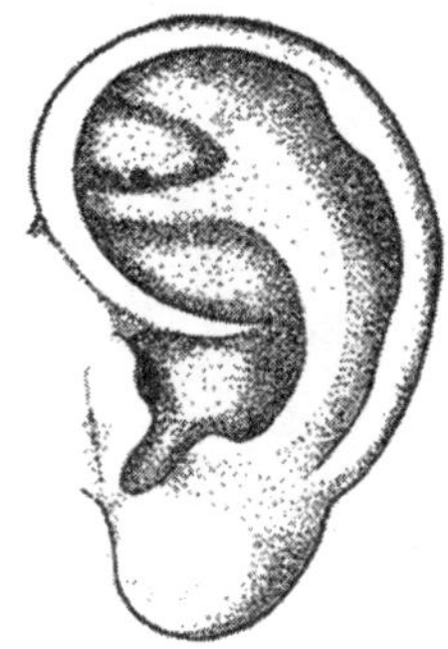

Bed Wetting

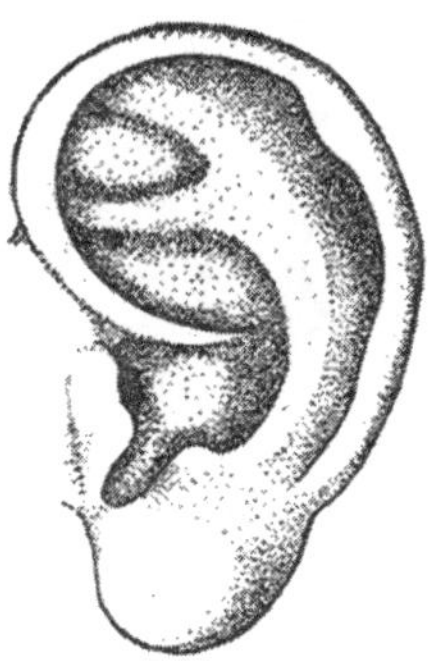

Constipation

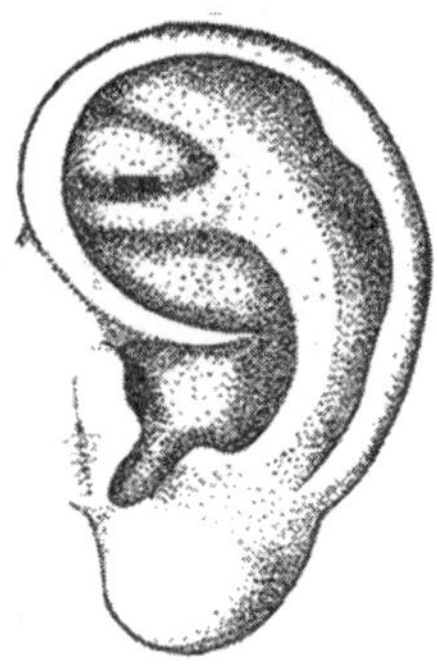

Blood Pressure

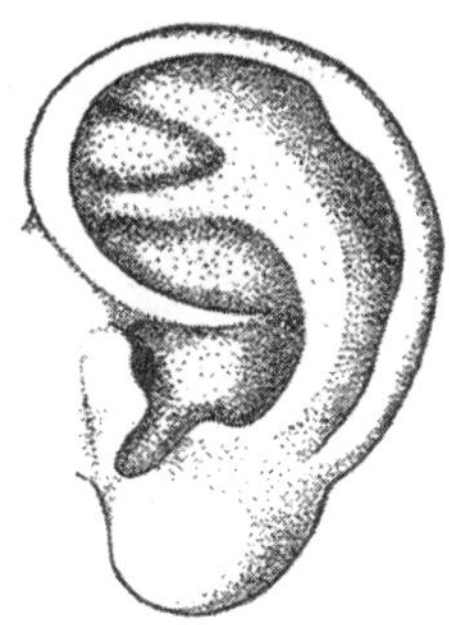

Insomnia

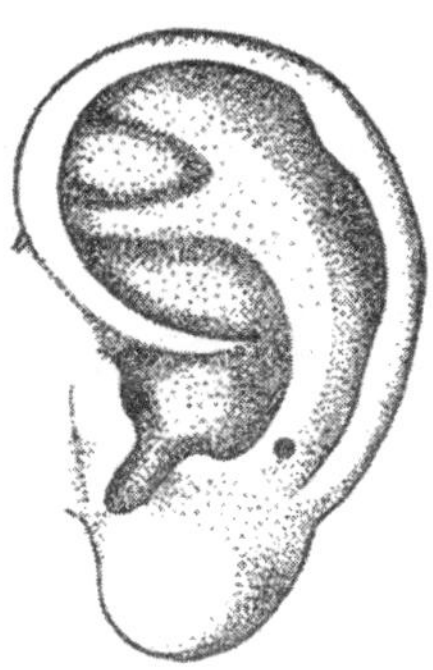

Diabetes

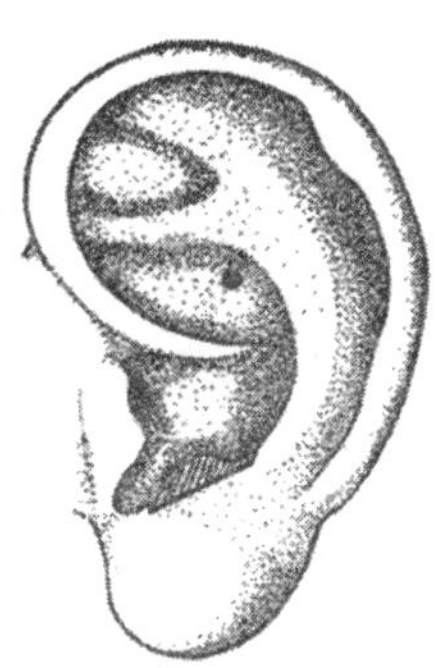

Impotence

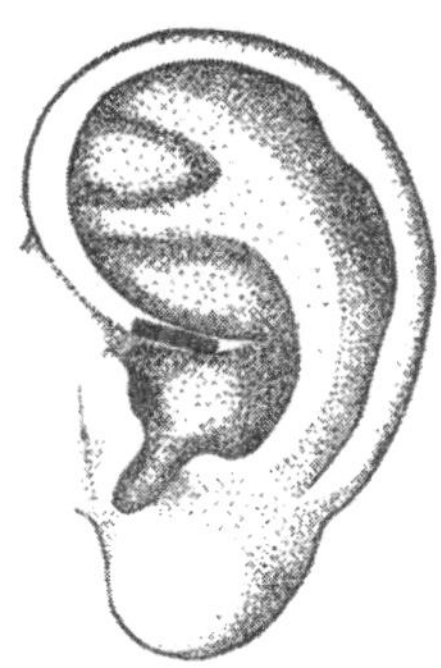

Appendix

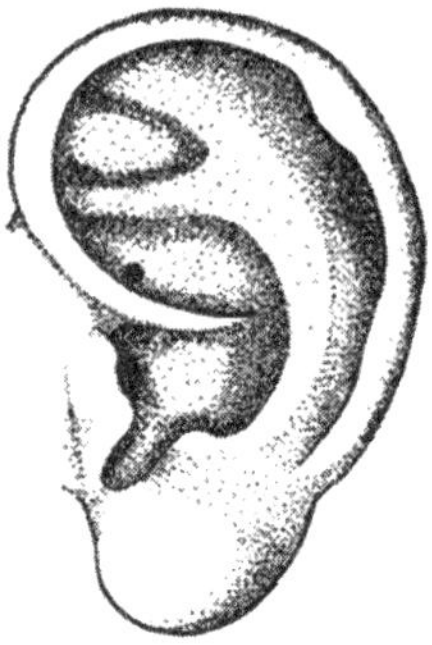

Asthma Attack

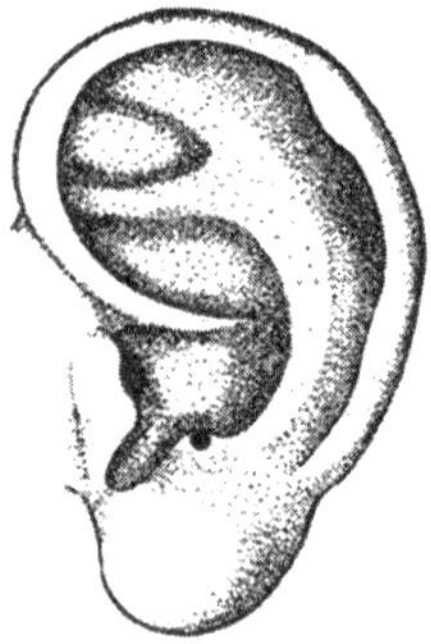

Stomach upset

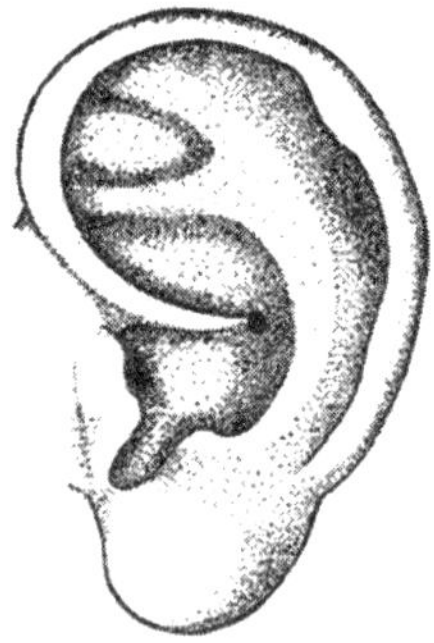

Urticaria

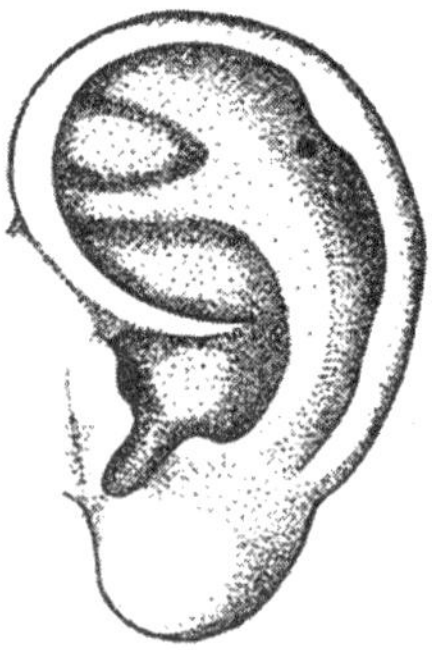

Tonsillitis

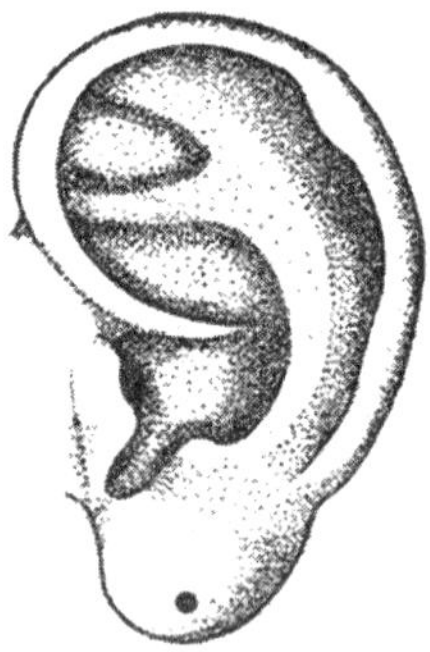

Vertigo

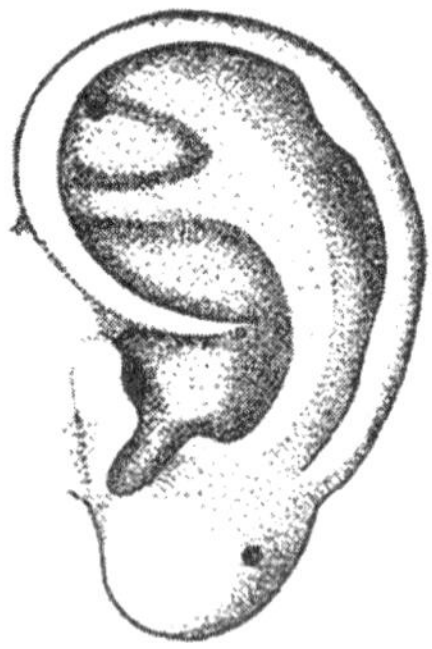

Hernia

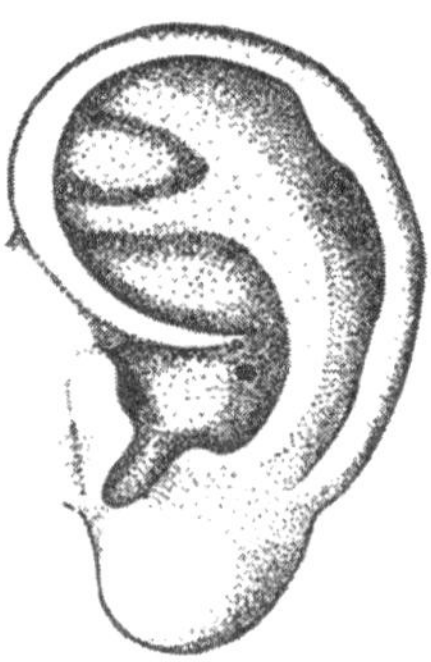

Concentration Improvement

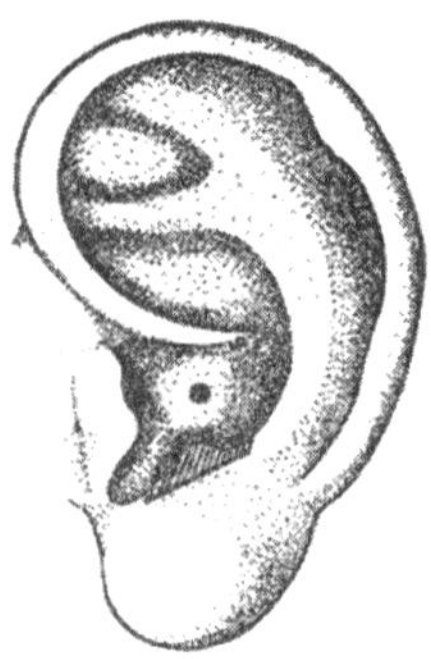

Sneezing bouts

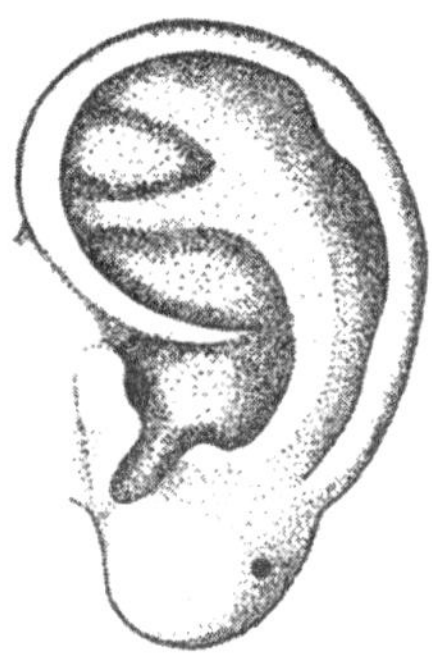

8

Case Histories

TREATING the body by auricle is a little known method in India. Hence the possibility of quoting extensive and varied cases through local experience is limited. However, with authenticity I can relate my personal experience at my clinical practice. Having treated by now thousands of patients by Acupuncture, ever since I learned this admirable, efficient and simple method of treatment, I have been using auricle for the first line of treatment both for diagnosing the body physiology and condition of various vital organs and also for treatment purpose. Invariably to the great surprise of the patients, in the first treatment itself the patient recovers visibly and at times in a major way even from long-standing pains and aches. The organ problems show clear pathology and recovery after treatment.

Few cases I have recorded here:

Fifteen years old Lumbago

I was practising in Gujarat. The patient was an NRI. The patient came to me stating he is staying in a cold place in England, he has been having this lower back pain for the last fifteen years.

TREATMENT

I traced the sensitive spot in his anti-helix close to lumbago point. As I started giving mild pressures with the probe the patient reacted with severe pain. I inserted in all four needles. One at the lumbago point horizontally, another at the thalamus point vertically, third at the shenmen and the last needle at the kidney point. The patient was asked to lie down for twenty minutes. Two needles at the lumbago and the thalamus were left *in situ* and the patient was asked to remove them after reaching home. Next day the patient reported very diminished pain. The treatment was repeated four times after which small seeds were taped to the point and the patient was asked to press it from time to time. A month later he reported from England his pain had completely gone.

Hiatus Hernia

The patient was a fifty-five year old lady. Thin and a bit emaciated. She was having swallowing problem for more than a year. It was diagnosed as hiatus hernia. It is the case when stomach lining goes into oesophagus. She was finding difficulty even to drink a glass of water comfortably. The solids were less of a problem in comparison to liquids.

TREATMENT

I found painful tender spots around oesophagus and cardiac orifice. Further her spleen was tender. I gave strong electrical stimulation with my hand-held electro stimulator machine in the area from mouth to cardiac orifice. Further Zero point and three needles horizontally facing the alimentary canal passage from mouth to cardiac orifice. The patient was asked to lie down for twenty minutes. The needles were removed and the patient was asked to drink a glass of water. To her astonishment immediately she could drink the water with ease. The treatments were repeated for six sittings to strengthen her system.

Vertigo

The patient, a gentleman of forty-eight years, reported he was having vertigo problem occasionally for past eight months with the frequency of two to three times a week.

TREATMENT

I gave him stimulation with a probe in internal ear point and triple heater point. Fixed seeds in the internal ear point and asked to press it from time to time. He reported a great relief in a week's time. After a month he again reported telling his vertigo problem had vanished.

Stomach Ulcer

The patient is a forty-year old slim medical representative. He had a severe case of duodenal ulcer for two years and was under medication which was giving him relief from time to time.

TREATMENT

On checking his alimentary canal route with the probe, I found his stomach and small intestine were affected. Apart from that his heart and triple warmer were very active. I sedated the heart and triple warmer and tonified kidney. Also treated his lung which was causing excess of dryness leading to ulcer. The balming sedative points, shenmen and zero point were applied regularly. It took him eight treatments of twenty minute duration each for results to filter in and to feel relieved. He continued the sittings for some more time to consolidate the results.

Dental Pain

It was the time I had started understanding ear reflexology. My mother has come to pay us a visit. One night she suddenly started having upper right molar tooth pain.

TREATMENT

I applied strong stimulation with a probe in the L-4 point for upper teeth in the lobe. The results were instantaneous. Her pain vanished. Later I applied some sedative points like shenmen and tranquilliser. Her situation stabilised and she started having faith in treatment by ear points.

Memory Problem due to Anxiety

It was examination time. My friend's daughter was getting panic syndromes. She ended up forgetting most of what she had studied in the examination hall. Her parents were now getting panic syndrome. They requested me to help her before her finals. She started taking ear acupuncture treatments.

TREATMENT

I treated initially in heart and shenmen in both the ears with four needles. After a few sittings I treated her adrenal, master cerebral and memory points. After about ten sittings she started feeling comfortable about exams. Much calmer, she not only faced the exams with calmness but did much better than her average performance in the finals as her concentration for studies also improved.

These are a few cases I have recorded here. As my clinical experience grows I have seen auricular therapy yields quick and lasting results both for pains and organ problems.

Cases Recorded World Over in Auriculotherapy

Ear is an admirable tool for detecting organ condition in the body and general condition of the body. It provides a more clear diagnosing tool in comparison to other traditional modes like pulse diagnosis and tongue diagnosis mainly due to the clarity in the findings.

The problem areas apart from being tender may show other signs like being discoloured, having dry or flaky skin, high conductivity by electro probe, etc.

Some of the established records are given below:

1. In 1995 at the international symposium on auricular medicine in China, case studies by practitioners showed ear reflex diagnosis is effectively used to detect — malignant tumors, coronary heart disease, pulmonary tuberculosis, colon and lung and uterine cancers, liver damage, etc.

- Colon cancer revealed dark red capillaries in superior conchae.
- Lung cancer revealed brown pin patches in inferior conchae area.
- Uterine cancer showed spotted depressions in the internal genital areas.
- Hepatitis showed clear reactive points around liver area.
- A dark red region around gall bladder area revealed the disease.
- Stomach and duodenum appeared shiny and red when infected.
- Many clinical cases were studied and statistical proof taken of several hundred patients.

(Reports from the journal, *Auriculotherapy* of Dr. Terry Oleson at UCLA Pain Management Centre — Los Angeles)

3. Ear Acupuncture is used extensively in South Asian countries like Korea, Hong Kong, Bangkok, Singapore and China for drug addiction and other substance abuses including food abuse leading to obesity. The results are good and lasting. (Excerpts from *Practical Ear Needling Therapy* published by Medicine and Health Publishing Co., December 1991, Hong Kong.)

   A 17-year-old student dying from a heavy heroin overdose was admitted in coma in the Army General Hospital in Bangkok. He was given Ear Acupuncture treatment by Dr Aroon. Ten minutes later the boy opened his eyes and tided over from emergency.

   Dr Aroon routinely cured every opium and heroin addict with acupuncture in 15 days, the exceptions being young addicts in teens who either lacked the necessary confidence in the cure or they were afraid of the needles.

Method of treatment : Dr Aroon inserts needle in the reactive spot of the ear, connects the needle with six volt electrostimulators for 30 minutes. In fifteen minutes the patient feels well, his dizziness and muscular aches gone. Dr Aroon initially repeats the acupuncture process two or three times a day for first three days and once daily afterwards for a minimum period of 15 days. The patient's recovery is stable and sustained.

3. **Acupuncture Anaesthesia**: This is another area, where routinely and extensively acupunture is used for bringing anaesthetic effect for surgery.

   The *Practical Ear Needling Therapy* reports 80,000 cases operated in Shanghai district of China alone. For this both ear and body acupuncture points are used combinedly. In such cases the post-operative care is minimum as the patient recovers fast with no drug inhibitory problem affecting the system.

   It is reported that in 100 cases of mitral commissurotomy performed under acupuncture anaesthesia, the patients did not have any drop in blood pressure and their recovery was swift.

   This also favours well with those who react adversly to drug anaesthetics and also in underequipped places as in this treatment the tools for anaesthesia are very simple and can be fitted in a pocket.

4. It is reported in Dr Terry Oleson's journal *Auriculotherapy* that this therapy facilitates the natural, self-regulating homoeostatic mechanism of the body by diminishing overactive bodily function or increasing underactive physiological processes.

5. From Prof. Dr Lohiya's experience as reported in *Advance Acupuncture,* published by Indian Academy of Acupuncture Science:

Dr Lohiya has an extensive experience in Acupuncture field in India having treated thousands of patients in numerous camps conducted by him in Maharashtra and also in his hospital at Aurangabad.

He states "Personally I rate ear acupuncture as the best microsystem of acupuncture. The results are excellent. Generally we add a couple of ear acupuncture points to our prescription of body acupuncture in almost every patient."

Some cases handled by Dr Lohiya:

1. One doctor whom I had needled at hip point told me that he had restricted hip movements for past six months and now he could perform all the hip movements without any pain.
2. A patient for hoarseness needled at throat point started speaking clearly and loudly after needling.
3. A lady doctor who was needled for mouth ulcers at the mouth point found the ulcers disappeared within couple of minutes.
4. During a camp in Mumbai a lady came for treatment of hypertension. Her B.P. was 230/130mm hg. The bleeding was done at the ear apex. The B.P. recorded after 10 minutes was 150/96mm hg.
5. A patient from Israel came for treatment for cigarette addiction. His shenmen, lung, mouth and internal secretion were needled. The patient was deaddicted after only two sittings.
6. A patient of acute congestive glaucoma was treated in the Hyderabad camp. The patient was brought by an ophthalmic surgeon. The surgeon had planned for enucleation as the patient was not responding to medicines. His ear apex and liver point were bled. Dark

red blood sprang from there. The intraocular tension was reduced in 5 minutes.

These are the cases as written by Dr Lohiya in his journal.

These above cases should sufficiently drive home the point that auriculotherapy or ear acupuncture is a hidden treasure in the medical science waiting to be tapped. What is admirable about it is for one it is drugless and the information can be grasped and made to use in most cost-effective manner with anyone with sufficient interest to understand and follow the method. It will be a boon to poor nations like ours if only this treasure is understood, valued and used.

Organ Map in the ear

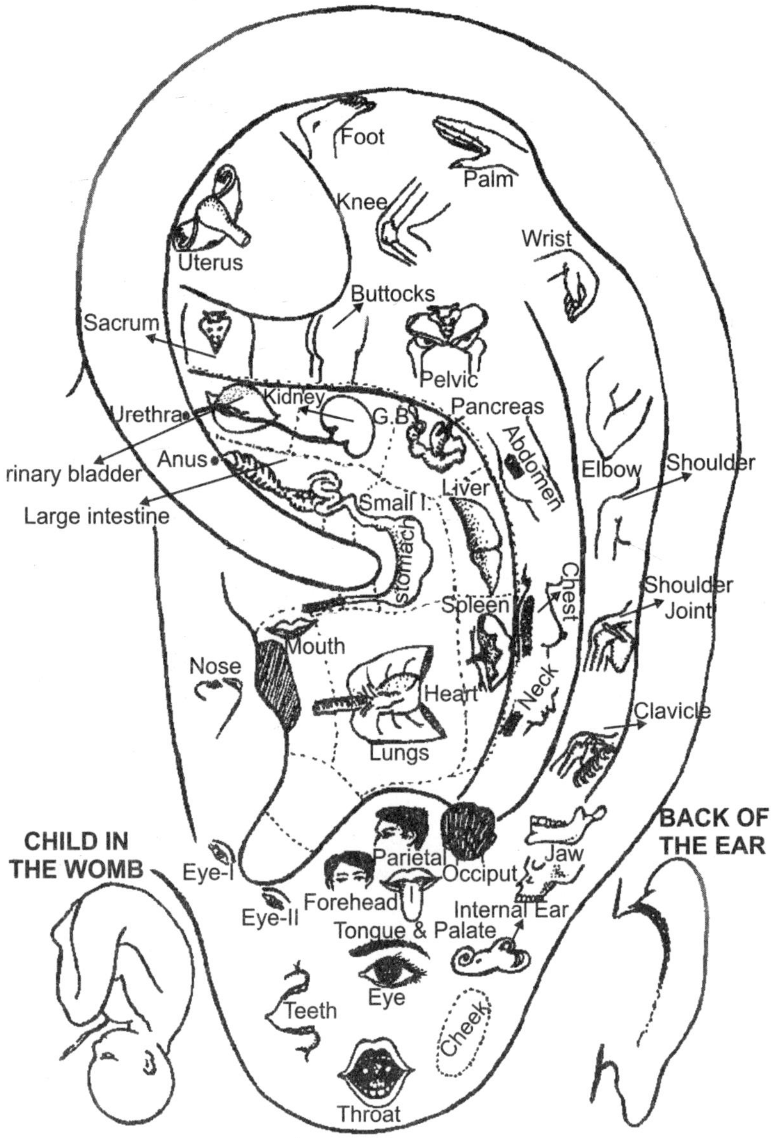